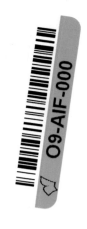

Dementia Reimagined

Dementia Reimagined

*Building a Life
of Joy and Dignity
from Beginning to End*

Tia Powell, MD

AVERY   *an imprint of Penguin Random House*   *New York*

AVERY

an imprint of Penguin Random House LLC
penguinrandomhouse.com

Copyright © 2019 by Tia Powell
Photo on page 61 photographer unknown. Permission to reprint
granted by Boston University Alumni Medical Library Archives.
Penguin supports copyright. Copyright fuels creativity, encourages diverse voices,
promotes free speech, and creates a vibrant culture. Thank you for buying an authorized
edition of this book and for complying with copyright laws by not reproducing, scanning,
or distributing any part of it in any form without permission. You are supporting writers
and allowing Penguin to continue to publish books for every reader.

Most Avery books are available at special quantity discounts for bulk purchase for sales promotions,
premiums, fund-raising, and educational needs. Special books or book excerpts also can be created
to fit specific needs. For details, write SpecialMarkets@penguinrandomhouse.com.

9780735210905 (hardcover ISBN)
9780735210929 (ebook ISBN)

Printed in the United States of America
10   9   8   7   6   5   4   3   2   1

Book design by Meighan Cavanaugh

For my mother and her mother, for my family, and for all those whose families are touched by dementia.

Contents

Dementia Reimagined

Chapter 1

De-'Men-Sha:
An Introduction

On a ferociously cold spring afternoon, I headed to Manhattan's Upper East Side for a concert in a church. It took a few minutes to find my way to the right room, where people filed into the rows, taking seats, cheerfully greeting family members and friends. The crowd was notably diverse, with quite a few older people, some little kids, hipsters, an elegant Latino family, a slightly disheveled man with shopping bags. We had assembled to hear the Unforgettables, a chorus for people with dementia and their caregivers. It was the inspiration of New York University researcher Mary Mittelman, who set out with the explicit intention to improve quality of life for those with dementia and those who care for them. By the appointed hour, the church was full of people and joyful anticipation.

The chorus worked its way through old standards, cheerfully led by Tania Papayannopoulou and Dale Lamb. We hailed the Chattanooga Choo Choo and left our hearts in San Francisco. We clapped along with great enthusiasm. Then one of the chorus members came right up front for a solo on "My Funny Valentine." She was a tall and stately blonde, beautiful now and surely devastating fifty years ago. She was an imperfect singer; she wielded the microphone tentatively and fell short on a few high notes. From one point of view, her solo was ill advised. From another, it was brilliant. Unbeknownst to her, a couple seated in the back row of the chorus had abandoned their seats and begun to dance together in the aisle, with delight and dignity. Perhaps this was their song. It was easy to imagine them dancing to "My Funny Valentine" when it was new and they were, too. He was tall, she was small; they looked happy and comfortable together. It was impossible to know which of them had dementia, not that it mattered at all. My eyes misted over, and I was not the only one.

Here is the thing: Dementia lasts for years. Most of that time, people with dementia retain the skills, memories, and passions that allow joy and inclusion in the larger social world, if we would but let them in.

A family story started me thinking about dementia some years ago. On an autumn day, two women sit together on a sunny screen porch in Washington, DC. They look alike; they are mother and daughter. Silver-haired and tiny, neither is quite five feet tall. One is in her sixties, one in her nineties. The younger woman radiates energy, bustling about, always the good daughter. She has managed to get the frail, mute older woman settled in a comfortable chair to enjoy the mild and lovely day. She arranges a rainbow-colored afghan, crocheted many years ago by the older woman, tucking it in around her. "There, Mother!" She beams. "How is that?" The older woman struggles to speak, which she has not done for months. The daughter waits. The silence is tremendous. The older woman produces a single word, a word that must stand for all she cannot say. Her eyes are fierce with effort. She whispers, "Lousy."

That was my grandmother's last word, spoken some months before she died of dementia, and long before my mother herself developed the dementia whose consequences would kill her.[1] I didn't know it at the time, but when my mother told me this story, it triggered a change in the way I understood dementia, a change that is ongoing. Like other serious diseases, dementia affects not only the person with the illness but all those whose lives touch hers.

My family has certainly felt the sting of dementia. I am a physician, but medical training never prepared me to address the challenges of dementia that I faced as a daughter and granddaughter. Having dementia or seeing a loved one suffer from it can be lousy, as my grandmother said. Millions of people across the globe can attest to that. But dementia isn't always lousy. Bad aspects can't be eliminated, but they can be diminished and compressed, making the experience *less* lousy for everyone.

My formal education in dementia started in medical school, though what we learned on the topic then, in the 1980s, was not enormously useful. We studied the different types, based on the initial symptoms or the type of brain pathology. Since there were essentially no treatments, the focus was on taxonomy rather than assistance. We were like eighteenth-century biologists, identifying different species of snails or butterflies, with no plan other than description. I learned about SDAT, or senile dementia of the Alzheimer type, about organic brain syndrome. Many of those categories have subsequently been renamed, redefined, combined, or eliminated altogether.

We also learned the basics of brain anatomy. In our first year, a professor projected a slide of a fleshy blob the size of a big shrimp and asked the class to identify it. I am not sure any of us got the answer—I certainly did not. The blob turned out to be the hippocampus; we each have two of these, resting on either side of and near the base of the brain. The name in Latin suggests they look like sea horses, but I never saw the family resemblance. I was taught that the hippocampus is crucial in the work of remembering. That much remains true, though plenty else I was taught is now out-of-date. Of course, that happens throughout medicine. Our current knowledge of cancer, of cystic fibrosis, of HIV provides a radically different and better understanding than was available decades ago. Still, even relative to other fields in medicine, our knowledge about how the brain works, what happens in neurons and brain networks—and how they break down— has exploded in the last twenty-five years.

But it is not only the technical, scientific understanding of dementia that is rapidly shifting. The most important change is our notion of where it sits in the arena of medical problems. A few decades ago, dementia was relegated to the back rows. There was nothing much to do about it, but more crucially, what would be the point? It was something that happened to old people and a few unlucky others. Surely it would make more sense to attack diseases that, if eradicated, would yield the survivors years of healthy life. If you fix something that affects only ninety-year-olds, your patient has a correspondingly brief life expectancy.

Medicine's view of dementia has undergone radical revision. Importantly, there are many more older people than there used to be, and since the risk increases with age, cognitive impairment is a concern for them all. Today there are more than 5 million people in the United States with dementia. That number will continue to grow as the population ages; in the United States, 10,000 baby boomers turn sixty-five every day. By the time a person reaches eighty-five, the chances of having dementia approach 40 percent.[2] Because of the cost of care, it is also one of our most expensive diseases, more than either cancer or heart disease. Dementia costs us about $200 billion yearly, a figure that includes both formal payment for care and an extraordinary amount of unpaid care.[3]

And here is more bad news: There is no effective cure or prevention, and none likely to arrive in the immediate future. That is one reason why dementia is the disease Americans fear most.[4] Recent major research trials can fairly be described as a series of unfortunate failures. It takes a new drug roughly twelve years to go from inspiration through testing in FDA-approved trials to market. Only a tiny percent of drugs successfully complete this process, either because most don't work or because they have side effects that make their risks greater than the benefits. With no *cure* in sight, our research efforts need to incorporate how to *care* for those who have and will develop dementia. We cannot neglect the millions whose comfort should be supported through better palliative treatment.

Medicine is a hierarchical field, and one that clings to a sense of masculinity, whether appropriate or not. Years ago, my two young children were waiting in line at summer camp. Two middle school boys in front of them were wearing towels over their swimsuits. One boy said to the other, "Dude, your towel is pink!" The other boy, flustered, answered, "Dude! It's *faded red!*" The answer: "Dude, it's pink." "DUDE—FADED RED!" The second boy felt his manliness under attack, and was willing to deny reality to defend himself. Medicine essentially makes the same denial. It sees itself as manly, offering heroic cures. But a great deal of what medicine offers patients is *care*—incremental, accommodating, feminine (if you stick with the outmoded metaphor). Yet medicine is too embarrassed to admit this. Care seems soft and unscientific; we'd prefer to hand out swashbuckling cure.

It could have gone another way. Medicine could have taken seriously the Hippocratic instruction to cure sometimes, treat often, comfort always. The dream of cure can push care to the lowest rung of the medical ladder. But though we have yet to find cures for many illnesses, including dementia, defining cure as success means viewing care as failure. For dementia in particular, we must do better. Setting up cure as the only goal, especially when it is linked to saving money, is bound to fail. We do not need science *or* compassion, but always both. We should fund science to try to dent the trajectory of dementia, and we must also care for those who are incurably ill today. We need care *and* cure.

Our view of dementia is changing, but it needs to change more. How we treat others, particularly vulnerable others, is part of what defines us as a society. When we hide demented elders because they look or act strange, when we fail to provide caring ways and places to live with dementia, we fail in important responsibilities. And yet people struggle with how to meet their obligations and find little guidance available. Should I lie to my father to get him to take medication? To get him to move out of the house where he has lived for decades but is no longer safe? Can we prevent those with cognitive impairment from driving, and if we do, how will we improve public transportation to better accommodate elders?

At one point in my life, I thought I knew something about dementia because I could recognize its symptoms and identify a hippocampus. But even as a doctor, I was not prepared when my mother developed the disease. I did not understand the options. I had to learn along with my siblings what sort of care she might need at any given stage and try to get that for her. I don't think we made terrible mistakes, but we made some. Our choices were difficult and the consequences were impossible to know in advance.

Dementia experts note a number of factors that make dementia care, especially at the end of life, both poor in quality and costly without benefit. When I think back over my mother's treatment, I see markers of less than ideal care: barriers to pain control, unhelpful transitions from hospital to nursing home to emergency room. Her journey through dementia was typical in many ways. It illustrates just how far we are from a system that respects those with dementia and their families. All across the country, families are facing similar choices, and they are struggling to find the right thing to do.

My mother was lucky in many ways. She grew up in a big Irish Catholic family in the suburbs of Washington, DC. She was bookish and shy. She always excelled in school, skipping a grade and finishing college first in her class. She married a good man who had gone to the same parochial school. (A 1935 issue of the church bulletin celebrated the children with highest marks in each grade, listing my father in eighth grade and my mother in fourth.) She had six healthy babies, now six healthy adults. She possessed a mysterious, renewable personal energy source. She marshaled her troops through homework, dog walking, piano lessons, sports practices, and rehearsals for school plays, and then she painted the furniture and fixed the toilets.

Not everything was easy. The late sixties were hard for a good Catholic woman, a time when teenage boys had long hair like Neanderthals and teenage girls went without bras like you-know-whats. They used bad language and questioned authority. My mother was bewildered. She embarked on a graduate degree in women's studies to see if she could figure out what was happening. She read, among others, Shulamith Firestone, who advocated the abolition of pregnancy and the nuclear family. My mother was appalled. But gradually things calmed down. Her children grew up and made better choices in hairstyles and lingerie. They got jobs, they married; chaos no longer reigned.

Decades rolled by. My mother's dementia came on gradually and late in life. By her mid-seventies, she had noticeable lapses in memory.

My father was still alive, and together they made a reasonably functional team, living most of the year in Florida. My father had cancer,
and he remained mentally sharp though increasingly weak. In contrast, as my mother's cognitive skills steadily declined, a lifetime of
physical activity kept her spry. She could ride her bike in their gated
retirement community, since the circular trails always led back to her
own apartment. When they set out for the grocery store, my mother
would drive. My father would tell her where to turn, where to park.
He would lean on the grocery cart and she would bird-dog items as he
directed. Sometimes he had to stay anxiously with the cart while she
brought the car around, but generally they got through their daily life
without major mishaps.

But then their system began to fail. As my father became weaker,
he couldn't always accompany my mother. Her cognitive deficits progressed. She got lost on her way to a doctor's appointment; she arrived
very late and beside herself with anxiety. She was badly shaken for days
after. Things were falling apart. It was time to change, but my parents
were angry with us for suggesting as much. We were frightened. We
couldn't keep them safe more than a thousand miles away from their
closest child. All six of us lobbied hard, in unison, for a parental return
to Maryland, where they had raised us; still had an apartment, doctors, and friends; and where two of my siblings still lived.

With some resistance and much assistance, my parents moved
back. My father got sicker. He enrolled in home hospice, and after a
time, he succumbed to cancer. A home health aide had moved in during my father's final illness, and she stayed on after his death to care
for my mother. Things did not go well. My mother was grieving and
her symptoms got worse. Once she ended up around the corner from
my sister's house in downtown DC and asked a stranger planting

tulips if my sister lived near there. My mother couldn't remember her daughter's married name, but the neighbor figured it out and pointed her in the right direction. The neighbor also ratted her out to my sister. We started to worry about her driving and finally got her to stop. She was extremely angry about giving up the keys. Hostile negotiations earned her a new nickname: the THWP, or Tiny Hibernian Warrior Princess.

My mother became paranoid. She lost small objects and blamed the aide. She began to stockpile pencils, since she believed the aide was hiding them to prevent her working on the crossword puzzle. Pencils were under the mattress, in the drawers, in the bathroom. In her prime, my mother cooked Thanksgiving dinner for twenty-five people with the tactical skill of a general going into battle. Now she was a risk in the kitchen, forgetting a pot on the stove or saving leftovers until they were blue and furry. Medication management became a problem. Knowing her memory was faulty, my rule-loving mother made an index card and taped it to her bathroom mirror. It said, "Take your medicines." And she did, over and over, until she became delirious from overdosing. Under protest, the index card was removed.

She had very little to do all day. Hours crawled by. My always active mother had no chores, no tasks to structure her lifelong productivity. The aide wanted to watch television; my mother didn't. They were not happy together. My sister found activity groups that helped a bit but didn't solve the problem. In one moment of comic relief, my Catholic mother went with my sister to the basement of a local synagogue that sponsored activities for those with dementia. My mother looked around at the nice ladies with Jewish names. She smiled tentatively. She spoke slowly, confiding to the ladies, "Some of my best friends . . . are synagogues." Laugh out loud or crawl out of the room? My sister was torn. But they took her revelation in stride and went on with bingo. Over time, my mother's theories about the pencils grew more elaborate, and the atmosphere at home grew more strained. Something had to give.

It came as a surprise to me that staying in one's home is not always the best option. For my mother, home had become a prison. My sister took her to visit an assisted living facility connected with a parish church and parochial school. My mother loved seeing the school kids trooping by. She would have more to do, people to talk to. She could dine with a group of silver-haired ladies each night, at a sweet round table with a tablecloth and a flower in the middle. She could bring some of her furniture, enough to fill her single room. She had few regrets leaving behind her apartment, her last independent dwelling. She was a great walker, even then, and could easily walk more than a mile. She enjoyed strolling around her new neighborhood, always accompanied, looking at the school, the old trees, the vegetable gardens.

Assisted living had its ups and downs. My mother flunked having dinner with the first group she was assigned to, since she introduced herself to everyone at every meal. They complained and she went to a different group, more obviously impaired. The staff was not unkind, but they were busy. My mother always preferred baths to showers—she loved nothing better than a relaxing "soaky bath." Although there was a bathtub available, it meant a worker standing by to make sure she was okay. It was easier for the staff if my mother showered in her own bathroom. Baths became a pleasure she would have to do without. This is what you can lose in moving to an institution, even one that tries to be friendly: They evolve to match the needs of those who run the place. What is fun or pleasing for residents may not make the top of anyone else's list.

. . .

Things rolled along for a year or so, until the next crisis. My mother had trouble breathing and went by ambulance to the hospital. A physician called me from the emergency room and asked whether they should try to resuscitate her heart if it stopped. I asked if she showed signs that her heart was likely to stop. He said no. I asked if he knew why she was short of breath, causing her trip to the hospital. He said no. I observed there was no way to know if her unidentified condition was easily treatable. He agreed. I said that her family would be happy to discuss resuscitation status when the need arose, but his call seemed premature. I wanted to know what the initial tests showed and what her doctors thought the matter was. He seemed a bit embarrassed. This too for me was a revelation. To this young doctor, my mother was an old woman with dementia and therefore not someone who should receive an ordinary evaluation for a common medical problem. How was he to know how we saw her, as someone who enjoyed her life, walked miles a week, had no particular physical ailments, and was a force of nature? Was he out of line? Or was I now one of those unrealistic family members who demand unhelpful treatment, increasing burdens and bringing no benefit?

The hospitalization was scary. My mother went to the ICU with an unusual blood disorder with the ominous name thrombotic thrombocytopenic purpura. I stayed overnight; she became increasingly confused and agitated, constantly trying to get out of bed and remove her tubes. I slept on and off, holding her hand, with my head on our hands to make sure she didn't sneak away. Late that night she had a seizure. A grand mal seizure is terrifying to watch, even when you have seen one before. Watching your mother have one is not an experience I recommend.

She returned to the assisted living facility, weaker and more cognitively impaired; she soon ricocheted back to the hospital. Now she had clots blocking the main arteries to her lungs, a consequence of her blood disease. We opted for a simple procedure, the insertion of a filter to keep clots from reaching the brain and causing a stroke. A kind physician who looked like a middle schooler came to her room and drew all over the whiteboard to explain the procedure. Since she was recovering from delirium—an acute state of confusion common in critically ill elderly people—and was suffering from dementia, it is entirely a fiction that she provided informed consent. Nonetheless, Doogie Howser said the appropriate words, and she smiled and signed the paper. No harm done. I was her surrogate decision-maker and thought the procedure was appropriate; I didn't insist on signing the form. But in hospitals all over the country, patients with limited understanding are agreeing to procedures that may not be in their best interest. Later that day, my mother proudly pointed out the doctor's diagram. There were lots of big loopy arrows that looked like the long ears of a basset hound. She told me the picture showed she'd given birth to a puppy and that was why she needed to stay in the hospital. I told her gently that she had a problem with blood clots. She looked put out. We went back to discussing events from her childhood. Her procedure went forward without a hitch.

This hospital stay marked the turning point from healthy demented person to a frail elder at risk for falling, both literally and metaphorically. My mother had almost never entered a hospital except to have babies, and now she'd had two serious admissions in short order. An enthusiastic walker just months before, she could no longer get from bed to chair. Never tall, she had become minuscule, a feisty leprechaun who might almost rest in the palm of your hand. She went to a rehab facility, where I came upon her working away like a terrier on the upper-arm bike, pedaling for all the world. Her arms and legs grew stronger, but her cognition did not. This is typical for a person with dementia. A frail brain at baseline makes it easier for a serious illness to harm cognition further. And that sparked the next transition. She was no longer welcome in her assisted living facility. She would need a skilled nursing facility.

My siblings who lived in Washington took on the lion's share of checking out nursing homes. Some were pretty to look at but seemed cold. Some were too far to visit regularly. One was small and attractive enough, but visitors were welcome only during a few hours daily, and upon arrival were kept in a windowless antechamber for what seemed like a long time. This lack of transparency gave the impression that things going on inside should not be seen, and that was a deal-breaker.

My father had been a successful attorney; they had saved so that my mother had funds to pay for nursing home care. But until we started looking, I had no idea the costs were so staggering. If you look up the average cost of a nursing home, you may find estimates of roughly $85,000 per year, but that is a deceptive number that typically reflects the rate that Medicaid pays. If you don't qualify for Medicaid or live in a higher-cost area—Anchorage, Alaska, is especially expensive—you may face annual costs nearly twice that amount.[5] A surprising number of people are under the impression that Medicare pays for long-term care. It does not. For those without assets, Medicaid will cover costs, though not every nursing home welcomes the lower Medicaid fees. People in the middle, with some assets but not enough to cover the crushing financial burden of long-term care, can "spend down" their assets until they qualify for Medicaid. There will be no inheritance for the family, and a surviving spouse may be in financial trouble, too. My mother's costs were covered by savings, but this level of expense is not feasible for most Americans. We lack an adequate national plan to cover the costs of care for the millions who will develop dementia in the coming decades. What I learned in medical school and in my training as a psychiatrist never prepared me for this.

My mother went to a memory care facility with a pleasant living and dining area, and a little garden you could see from the main rooms. Inexorably, she became weaker and more impaired. She could not walk independently. She could no longer dress or bathe or use the toilet. She could feed herself, but with substantial help and increasing difficulty. This is severe dementia, approaching the end stage of a fatal illness. She spoke less often, though she would beam at family members who came to visit. Once, as I spooned pudding into her mouth, I recalled feeding my children when they were small and thought about my mother feeding me. It felt both elemental and very sad.

My mother was happier than when she was less demented. She no longer elaborated complex paranoid theories about people hiding her pencils; she didn't have the bandwidth. She was content to be cared for and was mostly cheerful. But then she started to have odd spells in which she'd stare into space, shaking and speechless. She was evaluated for strokes and seizures, but nothing turned up. After one of these episodes, back in the ER again, a monitor showed heart block—the electrical system that controls the heartbeat was failing, causing ominous pauses. An excellent problem, for there is a solution. My mother needed a pacemaker.[6]

But not so fast. My grandmother had lived for twelve years with a pacemaker, and her own six children deeply regretted ever agreeing to it. My grandmother's dementia culminated in bed-bound immobility and muteness, and an apparent lack of joy. My mother had told us never to give her a pacemaker, and her siblings all felt the same. As far as advance directives went, my mother had done everything right. She formed an educated opinion about a specific treatment in a specific context and expressed that opinion in unambiguous terms on more than one occasion. She had a child who is a physician and bioethicist and appointed that child as a health care proxy.

Nonetheless, along came the cardiologist. He told my siblings that "no one is allowed to die of heart block." Also, no palliative care could be offered, since any symptom would come without warning and would be untreatable. He claimed that her death from heart block would feel "like drowning." He also noted that most cardiologists would refuse to turn off a pacemaker. He would consider doing so only if all six siblings agreed in writing. Not only could we lose the option of ceasing treatment if the cardiologist moved or changed his mind, but this last condition of unanimity was a way to override my mother's selection of a health care agent. Our family would be required to maintain her pacemaker if any one of us wanted it.

Even today I am angry at this doctor. Instead of helping, he made things worse. He was not able to say, "Think of this medical problem as one among many. How will what we do with her heart fit in with the overall goals of her care?" He didn't mean to be unkind. But doctors too often shrink their responsibilities to fit the size of their expertise. For older patients, who are likely to have many things going wrong at once, this is a disaster. He saw only a tree and missed the forest of my mother's serious medical problems.

My mother, though reluctant to comment, ventured: "Whatever the doctor thinks is best." Should we stay with her earlier wishes or go with her current passive neutrality? We had agonizing and anxious conversations, laced with dark humor. My brother said, "Whatever else happens, I am telling you right now I don't want a pacemaker." There was a brief silence. Then several of us spoke at once: "Oh, you are definitely getting a pacemaker!" "You'll get one if I have to put it in myself!" "I'm heading over there *right now.*"

We were joking, yet we were deadly serious. Most of my siblings thought it was a terrible mistake to consider a pacemaker, even if my mother did not currently object, but we were not unanimous. I felt I should be able to get the pacemaker shut down later, though I knew this could be a real challenge; the doctor had as much as said he would refuse. Surely all my training should allow me to provide this small service for my mother. Ambivalently, I agreed to the procedure, promising to find a way to have it turned off when the time came.

Some days later, the cardiologist showed up at my mother's bedside, shower cap on his head. Two of my siblings were there with her. "What are you doing here?" asked my mother. "I've come to take you for a pacemaker." "I don't want a pacemaker. You doctors do too much stuff to old people." My siblings asked my mother the same question in as many ways as they could. "Do you understand you might not live as long without the pacer?" "Yes. I've lived a good long time." And so forth. The pacemaker was canceled.

My mother was placed in hospice care at the nursing home so she would not be subjected to ER visits with every episode of heart block. The episodes would last for a few seconds with a complete loss of consciousness, leaving no memory behind. She had no fear ahead of time, no pain during, no memory after. She did not suffer, in sharp contrast to the cardiologist's prediction.

Then late one night my mother developed a slow heart rate, sweating, and shortness of breath. Hospice care at the nursing home was well intentioned but poorly organized. These clinicians should have had on hand the morphine and perhaps oxygen my mother would need, and they did not. No supplies could get there until the next morning, many hours away and likely after her time was out. My brother rushed to her side. She was transferred to the emergency room one last time, where she received the necessary oxygen and morphine, though lying on an uncomfortable gurney and not in her bed. She should have been spared this last, wholly unnecessary transition. She slept a good deal of the time. And then she was done. My mother did not die of dementia, as her mother had. She died *with* dementia, but *of* heart disease.

If my mother had received that pacemaker, she might have lived longer to die of dementia, just as she had not wanted. Medical technology comes attached to an engine that propels it toward patients. Unlike the vast majority of older people in America, she had six adult children to help her and we still stumbled our way along, trying our best, making mistakes. Yet she was one of the lucky ones. My family learned the hard way about caring for someone with dementia. We faced hard choices large and small, about what care we want for ourselves and how we ought to treat others.

This book is for all those who face dementia. You will see the disease more clearly, and this knowledge will make it less, not more, frightening. This book is about how hard it is to get things right—to plan, to get the right care at the right time, to pay for that care, and to work together to find better treatments and support. It tells you some of what you can do to make the experience of dementia a little less lousy and a bit more joyful. This illness is not just about loss; it is also about preservation—of affection, of dignity, of hope. You will learn how to make dementia less scary for someone you love, and for yourself.

Chapter 2

Invisible

Here is a paradox: In the past, dementia was invisible. At the same time, we looked right at it. How is this possible? People with all the symptoms of dementia were there, and those symptoms are responses to specific types of damage to the brain. But we had no category to capture those changes. They did not add up to an illness. Medicine had yet to bundle those symptoms into a concept of a specific disease, with expected changes and a predictable trajectory.

If Grandpa got lost on his own farm or threatened a beloved grandchild, friends and family noticed, of course. But they had no clear notions of cause or response to those disturbing changes. What we see now as dementia was taken long ago as just madness—not a specific illness but a chaotic falling apart. Think, for instance, of Jonathan Swift, who lived from 1667 to 1745 and died of dementia. He had friends and enemies in his time, but all agreed he was among the most brilliant and prolific writers of the day. Then his fine mind declined shockingly. He himself predicted this by looking up at a great oak and saying, "I shall be like that tree. I shall die at the top."[1] Older accounts of his later life describe him as "insane" or "mad."[2] But what was this madness?

Swift, a keen, even merciless, observer of the human condition, did not spare himself from scrutiny, as Leo Damrosch documents in his fine biography.[3] In 1738, Swift wrote, "I have been many months the shadow of the shadow of the shadow, or etc. etc. etc. of Dr. Swift— age, giddiness, deafness, loss of memory, rage and rancor against persons and proceedings . . ." He tallied up symptoms of dementia and even connected them with deafness, only recently recognized as a significant risk factor for cognitive decline. Swift left off depression, but this also was his lot:

> I have been very miserable all night, and today extremely deaf and full of pain. I am so stupid and confounded that I cannot express the mortification I am under both in body and mind [. . .] I hardly understand one word I write. I am sure my days will be very few; few and miserable they must be.[4]

Despite his prediction, Swift lived five more years. He had funds and friends and servants who saw to his care, but he lost the ability to recall their names; he could not feed or dress himself. He had to be "put to bed like the youngest child."[5] He stopped speaking. By the time he was seventy-five, an appointed committee declared him incompetent, finding that "he was of such unsound mind and memory that he is incapable of transacting any business or managing, conducting, or taking care either of his estate or person."[6] Swift's contemporaries looked at him and saw madness. Today we look and see dementia.

Those who shared Swift's malady but had no family, no money, and no connections did not receive the same care. In Swift's day, there was no notion that health care was due to every person who suffered. It was a comfort for purchase. Dementia in the poor, in those without families, went untreated and unseen.

Today we—society, families, people with dementia, doctors, scientists, policymakers—look at people with a similar constellation of problems and see a major public health challenge. The way we have defined dementia, both its nature and treatment, have changed radically over time. How we ought to care for those with the disease and what we owe to everyone who suffers from it remain open questions.

The history of our cultural response to dementia is not pretty. Looking back over the centuries, we find those with dementia in jail, in workhouses, in shackles, and in mental institutions. We have punished rather than treated. We have shown those who need help that they are a nuisance, a bother. The help that was offered in centuries past was designed to chastise, control, and minimize the trouble for minders while the inmates waited for death. Even today, we find those with dementia in our jails and homeless shelters. The way a society treats people with dementia creates a portrait of that society. In looking at how we respond to them, we see ourselves.

But there has long been a radically different response, running alongside the cruelty and indifference. For centuries, there have been those who care for and comfort those with dementia, who have seen their suffering and responded with compassion. Though they have no cure, they honor these people. They do not punish; they do not beat or starve. They don't tie anyone up. Whether family members or health professionals, they embody the Hippocratic aphorism: Cure sometimes, treat often, comfort always. Cruelty and comfort have been competing elements in the response to dementia, both in the past and still, less obviously, today. At times one, then the other, dominated; both were almost always there.

Today we are tackling dementia with a plethora of health policies, programs, dollars, and struggling families. But we have wasted so much time. We have pursued strategies that have not paid off. We have doggedly stuck with those strategies long after we saw them failing. We have argued about whether dementia arises from biological or social factors, when the plain truth is that like most illnesses, it is the product of both. We still don't have good answers for how to prevent, treat, or cure it. We are beginning to learn how to care for those with dementia, but far too few have access to good care. It has taken a long time to see dementia clearly, and we still have a long way to go.

We are going to look back into the past, so let's agree on what we're searching for. It's harder than you might think. Dementia is not a single illness, but a collection of illnesses, like cancer. Today we recognize multiple types of dementia with different causes and changes in the brain. Alzheimer's disease is one form, as are frontotemporal dementia and vascular dementia, and dementia associated with Parkinson's or Huntington's or AIDS. All share the common feature of irreversible cognitive decline, yet vary in the prominence of symptoms like memory loss or hallucinations.

The benchmark definition is the technical, medical one in the *Diagnostic and Statistical Manual of Mental Disorders,* fifth edition (*DSM-5*), psychiatry's bible of diseases affecting the brain. Here is a synopsis of Major Neurocognitive Disorders:[7]

> Significant cognitive decline from previous function in attention, executive function, learning and memory, language, perceptual-motor, or social cognition, based on:
>
>> Concern of the individual, someone who knows the person well, or the clinician;

Substantial impairment documented by neuropsychological testing;

Cognitive deficits that interfere with independence in everyday activities like paying bills or managing medications.

That gives us the basics and also shows why it's going to be hard to track down dementia in history. First, it doesn't even use the word *dementia,* but instead talks about *neurocognitive disorders,* a term unknown to speakers of plain English. If a doctor said you suffered from major neurocognitive disorder, a reasonable response would be "What the heck is that?" We'll encounter the same problem in the past; each age uses different names. At least today's experts have agreed on what *they* will call dementia, even if it's not the word the public uses. For a long time, there was no such agreement; doctors used a bewildering variety of terms for what they saw, which might or might not be what we call dementia.

The second problem with the *DSM-5* definition is that it is bloodless. It captures none of the experience of having dementia or caring for someone with it. Below the definition, *DSM-5* notes that depression, anxiety, agitation, hallucinations, paranoia, and wandering can all be part of this illness. These are the problems that brought such sorrow to Jonathan Swift and to my mother. If you care for someone with dementia, these features are the ones that make life with dementia tough, that mean your loved one may no longer be able to stay at home or in the assisted living facility. For you, these features are not an afterthought.

So here's how we'll recognize dementia: a syndrome of decreasing cognitive function that shows up as problems in memory, learning, speaking, planning, and even moving. Most people with dementia are old, but not all. Anxiety, depression, agitation, and paranoia are common. The course is irreversible, the prognosis fatal.

Suppose we borrow a time travel device, something like Mr. Peabody and Sherman's WABAC machine. We'll investigate what people in the past saw when they looked at someone with dementia. We'll have to check out a dizzying array of names—like senility, dotage, and fatuity. We'll have to watch out for other illnesses that used to be called dementia, but are not what we're looking for. Schizophrenia, an entirely different illness, was once known as dementia praecox, loosely translated as dementia in the young.

It also won't be easy to find old people with dementia in the past. The average life-span in the United States didn't rise above the fifties until after 1900,[8] although the phrase *average life-span* is misleading. Infant mortality rates were abysmally high and helped pull down the average age. But if a child made it through the gauntlet of life-threatening genetic and infectious diseases, his or her chance of surviving to adulthood vastly improved. Unfortunately, there were still lots of other ways to die. A heart attack, a stroke, cancer, childbirth, or a fall from a horse were far more likely to kill then than now, and all of these also held down the average age. Of those relatively few who made it to old age, some had dementia.

There are ancient references to what we might call dementia. The ancient Greek physician Aretaeus labels "dotage" as "the calamity of old age, for it is a torpor of the senses, and a stupefaction of the intellectual faculties . . . Dotage commencing with old age never intermits, but accompanies the patient until death."[9] Cicero offered advice that makes sense today: "It is our duty to resist old age; to compensate for its defects by a watchful care; to fight against it as we would fight against disease . . . much greater care is due to the mind and soul; for they, too, like lamps, grow dim with time, unless we keep them supplied with oil."[10] Historian Karen Cokayne unearths this first-century quote from Roman poet Juvenal:

> But worse than all bodily ills
> Is the senescent mind. Men forget what their own servants
> Are called, they can't recognize yesterday's host at dinner,
> Or finally, the children they begot and brought up.[11]

Cokayne points out that the word *dementia* is used loosely in Latin, without differentiating between mental illness generally and an affliction of the aged.[12] Indeed, the building blocks of dementia are *out of* and *mind*; the word itself does not distinguish among different forms of losing one's mind. As we saw with Jonathan Swift, dementia was often lumped in with mental illness, a category so broad it included depression, epilepsy, and even having a child out of wedlock.

So not only will we need to seek dementia under multiple names, we'll need to unearth it in unlikely hiding places, including all those used to corral the mentally ill. But, some of you will say, dementia is not a mental illness. That turns out to be a complex issue, as ways of aggregating different brain diseases have also changed drastically. At the time we'll start our search, all brain diseases were part of the undifferentiated forest called madness.

Those who were viewed as mad shared a harsh fate, but why? Perhaps because of remnants of the medieval belief that mental illness meant possession by the devil. Because the devil was a powerful and crafty foe, powerful weapons must counter such evil. "Swingeing" (whipping), beating, starving, chaining, drowning—all were "treatments" aimed at the mentally ill. Through the seventeenth century, women who behaved erratically could be condemned as witches, with the penalty of beheading or burning. Fatalities were not the fault of the perpetrator, but a sign that the devil's strong grip was incompatible with life.

Many treatments for mental illness relied on water, perhaps because of associations with the moon, tides, and the waxing and waning of psychiatric symptoms. Sometimes a local spring was renowned for healing powers. Supplicants might go there, perform rituals, and sleep by the spring overnight, hoping to be well by morning. That sounds pleasant enough, but variations on the water theme included full immersion, sometimes known as dunking or "bowsening." A Scottish newspaper reported twice yearly dunking of lunatics at midnight in Lochmanur, as late as 1871.[13]

Punishment was the norm, not the exception. Certainly this was true at London's Bethlehem Hospital, or Bedlam, the oldest facility in Europe dedicated specifically to mental illness, having served that purpose since at least 1400. Today the hospital is a respected center for research, but back in the 1500s, Bedlam was rife with scandals. It is difficult to assess motivations from centuries ago, but it is hard to believe the keepers of the mentally ill understood their interventions as anything other than punishment, since beating, starvation, and near-drowning were frequently used as such. Blistering was painful and common, and consisted of placing heated glassware atop the skin to create blisters and draw out corrupting matter. Those with dementia were easily swept up in that response.

Let's focus on the new nation of the United States, and look to Britain as well, which shaped early American medicine and science. This period in American history is defined by radical change in every domain. America, breaking away from the British empire, could not contain its energy. There was ferment everywhere. Its borders pushed out. Settlers headed west in waves, starting farms and seeking gold.

Whole families and communities left home with the dream of owning land and carving out an independent life. Demand for land for these settlers fueled bloody and protracted conflict with the indigenous peoples. The destruction of Native American people and culture was viewed by settlers not as a tragic conflict, but as the triumph of civilization over savagery. America built and expanded, aggressively clearing the land of any obstacles to progress, whether trees or people.

Waves of immigrants came to the New World. Europe sent not only Protestants from England, but Catholics from Ireland and Italy and Jews from Germany and Russia. The slave trade brought captive Africans, if they survived the grueling conditions of the middle passage. Immigration from China and the rest of Asia ramped up early in the nineteenth century. Railways went west, built by Chinese immigrants under slave-like conditions.

Among all this ferment, all this bold expansion, how did an older person with dementia fit in? She didn't, really. Her portrait was left out as the bustling nation created its image. This was no time to be frail. Protecting the weak was not a priority; clearing places for the strong was the goal. Immigrants, given the rigors of travel, were generally young and healthy. Old people stayed behind in old countries. Families heading out to the dangerous frontier faced enough trouble without packing up confused elders for the trip. Small children fell routinely to fatal epidemics of infectious disease. Women died in childbirth. These were more important problems than cognitive deterioration in weak old people.

Many societies, ours included, like to believe they treat elders with respect. History, however, offers a decidedly mixed picture. Always, those with wealth and devoted families fared better, though not necessarily well. With funds and a family, you might remain comfortably in a private home, far from prying eyes and perhaps with kindly attendants. Families of more modest means stretched resources to include a frail, demented elder. The development of difficult behaviors might outstrip those resources, and the family would then seek some other placement. Then as now, those with dementia face a kind of sliding scale. With ample support and quiet, mild symptoms, home remains an option. As financial or human resources dwindle and symptoms like agitation or aggression overwhelm caregivers, expulsion becomes more likely.

If someone with dementia attracted notice, it was as an annoyance, a nonspecific management problem. They disappeared into an undifferentiated mass of those who had problems and caused problems.[14] Those who were elderly, poor, and demented might get the same begrudging treatment offered to amputees, single mothers, alcoholics, or the unemployed. Americans' earliest efforts to deal with people with dementia were to lump them together with others who couldn't care for themselves. If the family couldn't keep them at home, they went to the poorhouse or jail.

Perhaps it seems strange to throw those with dementia in jail. But it is not unusual to batch undesirables together. That is why the ghetto was invented in fifteenth-century Venice, then a great mercantile empire, drawing people from all over the world. Among those people were Jews, who were required by law to live within a small, crowded, and strictly delineated section within the city. Why not? They were all the same; they were all Jewish. But of course they were not remotely all the same. Jews came to Venice from Spain, Africa, Sicily, and Constantinople. They had different languages, dress, foods, and even liturgies. But all these differences were ignored; instead this group was seen as having a single identifying feature, and nothing else needed to be known of them.[15] That is how a ghetto works. It is not only a place but also a way of rendering individuals invisible. In a sense, this is also how many contemporary nursing homes work.

The poorhouse was one early type of ghetto. In the 1800s, poverty outweighed features like age, illness, and disability, and the poorhouse provided the bare minimum of shelter and food. Shame was a feature, not a bug. That there were hardworking poor who stayed out of the poorhouse proved, at least to some, that poverty was deserved—even chosen—and a direct result of sinful behavior. Appealing or even clean and safe conditions would only undermine efforts to reform residents from sins like sloth, gambling, and alcohol. The poorhouse pushed together those with physical and mental disabilities, the aged and the young, and those who were able-bodied but unemployed. This was no safety net, but a spiteful imitation of charity.

America set up poorhouses, which existed in the United States in diminishing numbers into the twentieth century. An impoverished older person with dementia might also land in jail, though criminal justice relied less on incarceration in America's early years. Those found guilty of severe crimes went straight to the gallows—no need for prison. For lesser offenses, outraged villagers might run a criminal out of town or sentence him to the stocks. This last punishment doubled as entertainment, as neighbors threw rotten vegetables at the publicly displayed miscreant.[16] In many states, laws gave local officials the authority to jail those deemed insane. There was no limit to the sentence, and jailed patients had almost no rights. They were condemned to dank, dark cells, with minimal food, clothing, and warmth.

The U.S.'s first psychiatric beds appeared in Pennsylvania in the 1750s, after a petition to the state assembly for the "cure and treatment of lunaticks."[17] Bedlam's methods prevailed, with blistering and shaving the scalp; the blacksmith was billed for "legg chains." State coffers were augmented by inviting the public to come gape at inmates for a fee. And things got pretty lively:[18]

> August 28, 1758, admitted AD, an Outrageous Person . . . January 27, 1759, Escaped Jno. Jones, a Lunatic; he forced Barrs of his Cell in ye night and fled without Notice . . . Thomas Dougan, a Lunatick, taken up upon the Streets naked the 20th inst. Said to come from ye East Jerseys.

New York Hospital converted space for the mentally ill in the 1790s, but it was hardly designed for comfort. The few unpainted, unheated cells in the basement "became so imbued with filth that they are exceedingly offensive."[19] A sensitive medical student records his "dismal reflections" in a diary, questioning the wisdom of treatments like "unexpected plunging into cold water . . . bleeding, purging, vomiting, streams of cold water on the head, blisters."[20]

Treatment took a step forward with the efforts of Benjamin Rush, whose profile adorns the logo of the American Psychiatric Association. Rush was a professor at the University of Pennsylvania when he published *Medical Inquiries and Observations Upon the Diseases of the Mind* in 1812.[21] He rejected theories linking madness to diseases of the liver, spleen, and intestines, and shunned notions of possession by the devil. He argued that it was a disease of the brain's blood vessels—a theory with surprising echoes in contemporary research. He was a man of science; he looked for physical root causes. Still, like many in the nineteenth century and since, he couldn't separate the moral from the biological. He fretted about moral causes of insanity, particularly onanism, or masturbation.[22] Excess use of the imagination might also cause insanity, he wrote, explaining why there are more mad poets and musicians than chemists and mathematicians. Other bad influences included poor climate, infidelity, atheism, and strangely, laughter, "a convulsive disease," which he claimed had killed an unnamed pope who "had seen a tame monkey put on part of his pontifical robes."[23]

Rush comes near to but never quite captures dementia in his observations. He listed many causes of memory loss, including intemperance in eating and drinking, "excess in venery" (lust), and fevers. He claims that one Sir John Pringle recovered his memory by quitting the use of snuff. In his long list, though, he never mentions old age. Illnesses he does describe include the afflictions of "demence," defined as an acute flightiness of ideas, and "fatuity," a state of "total absence of understanding and memory . . . slobbering, lolling of the tongue, and ludicrous gestures of the head and limbs."[24] Neither of these is what we recognize as dementia.

Some of Rush's observations stand the test of time. He argued that indiscretions with alcohol and overeating might lead to poor function in old age, a commonsense observation supported by contemporary evidence. Despite these tantalizing hints, though, he did not observe any illness that comes close to our contemporary notion of dementia.

Back in England, reform-minded Quaker Edward Wakefield visited Bedlam,[25] where he saw therapies based on second-century Greek physician Galen's theory of the four humors. Galen believed that all illness derived from an imbalance of body fluids, or humors. Treatment "balanced" fluids through bloodletting, starvation, purging, and the induction of vomiting. Wakefield's investigations found these ancient treatments, plus punishment, were Bedlam's main approach to mental illness. Restraints, especially chains, were the norm. Wakefield discovered a ward for women, each chained by an arm to the wall and given only a blanket for clothing. The men's ward used chains on legs as well as arms.

His subsequent report inspired Parliament to reform treatment of the insane. Wakefield built on the writings of earlier Quaker reformer William Tuke, who had stated that "The non-resistant principles of the Society of Friends were simply applied to modify the government of the insane from . . . one of fear, to a policy of gentleness."[26] This marks the beginning of *moral treatment*, which set aside bloodletting and chains in favor of compassion. It called for socialization between patients and attendants, the better to model calm, respectful, and rational behavior. Moral treatment creates a view of the mentally ill as "human beings suffering a terrible affliction, toward whom it is a duty to extend consolation, compassion, and kindness."[27] This was a radical departure indeed. It is nearly impossible to grasp today how shockingly these proposals—with care and compassion at their core—departed from the standards of the day.

When New York Hospital sought to modernize its mental health treatments in 1811, they turned toward moral treatment, and asked the advice of Samuel Tuke, William's grandson. Tuke's response catalogues the dos and don'ts of the approach. Do offer warm baths, especially to melancholics; provide a "liberal supper," especially to promote sleep in those with insomnia.[28] Don't provide "nauseous draughts," opium, bleeding, purgatives, or a "low diet" without calories or protein. Tuke urged his colleagues to "treat patients with uniform kindness and never deceive them." He found that walks in the country stilled the anxious mind and that "close confinement is of all things the most unsuitable." He stressed that "neither chains nor corporal punishment have ever been allowed on any pretext at the Retreat."

Among his major American proponents was Dr. Thomas Kirkbride. Like the Tukes, he was a Quaker, and an important link in the chain of Quakers who insisted on respect and nonviolence in the treatment of the mentally ill. Kirkbride was beloved of his colleagues, who fondly recalled his "countenance highly expressive of benevolence and

warmth of heart."[29] He was also an impressively capable administra-
tor. Taking on clinical leadership at the Pennsylvania Hospital when
he was only thirty-two, he adopted sweeping changes. He instituted
annual reports of statistics on the number and outcome of patients
treated. He believed that transparency was a hallmark of a well-run
and ethically sound institution, and would "break down ill-founded
prejudices" about mental hospitals. He banned bloodletting and other
"depleting" measures, setting aside the four humors for a more scientific and modern approach. He urged others to adopt these methods,
and helped found what eventually became the American Psychiatric
Association, the first national medical society in the United States. He
obtained the ample funds needed for high staffing ratios and the careful separation of patients so that vulnerable residents were not subject
to violence from physically aggressive ones. He trained his staff exten-
sively and in turn demanded high standards of them, asking that they
continually reflect on what sort of treatment they would want for
themselves or a loved one, and that they provide that level of kindness
and patience.

In a policy that represented a hallmark of moral treatment, Kirkbride strictly limited the use of restraints. In drafting "Rules and Regulations" for the Pennsylvania Hospital for the Insane, he noted that
"the use of restraining apparatus is productive of so many such serious
evils, and is now so nearly abolished in all well-conducted institutions
for the insane, that it will not be permitted to be applied here in any
case, except by the express direction of the physician of the institution."[30] The annual report of 1848 noted proudly that there was "no
reason for applying even the milder kinds of apparatus in a single one
of the 238 cases under care."[31]

Kirkbride took the high road on a debate that has lasted into the
present day—indeed, we are still struggling to curb the use of restraints.

It is painful to study the nineteenth-century argument. In the pages of the *American Journal of Insanity*, one superintendent wickedly satirized moral treatment, with its claim to "domicile your madmen and imbeciles in cozy cottages, with pleasant outlook and garden privileges [. . . and] employ only educated saints in sufficient numbers for companions, teachers and comforters."[32] He defended the infamous "Utica crib," a device that confined a mentally ill person within a webbing-covered bed, preventing sitting up and most forms of movement. Not surprisingly, it often came down to money. In the same journal, Dr. Ray of Maine noted the greater number of attendants required, and thus the far greater expense, for an institution that does not tie up the patients.

Almost 150 years passed before regulations to limit restraints gained ground in American mental institutions, hospitals, and nursing homes. (The UK already had such restrictions in place for generations.) A speedier change would have spared thousands untold misery and prevented no small number of deaths. I don't ignore the legitimate question of how to protect an agitated person—and her attendants—which remains controversial, even today. A frightened person is a dangerous person, as when a drowning swimmer pulls under the rescuer. As a psychiatrist, I have seen this danger firsthand.

Years ago, still in my internship year and fresh from medical school, I rotated through Creedmoor, one of New York State's public psychiatric facilities. The campus was vast, full of mostly empty squat brick boxes. This was during the period of deinstitutionalization, when as many patients as possible had been pushed out of the hospital. Those remaining included severely and chronically ill people who had been hospitalized for years and had no other options. One evening I worked the four P.M. to midnight shift and was called to see an agitated patient. When I arrived, a security guard and a nursing supervisor were waiting outside the locked unit door. I heard a rhythmic pounding, like a giant piston smashing a pylon into rock. Through the small glass pane, I peered far down the hallway. It was empty but for one enormous man. In my memory he is a colossus, his arm as big as all of me. He was methodically slamming a heavy metal door with such force that each time it hit the jamb, before bouncing back, large splotches of paint fell off the door and onto the floor. I thought, irrelevantly, *I didn't know you could slam a door so hard the paint fell off.* I then thought, *If he slams me that hard, I'll need more than new paint.* The security guard told me the patient had been at this a while, and that the nurses were trapped in the nurse's station. Sure enough, at the very end of the corridor was a glass-walled bunker. Two solemn women stared back at us, their eyes like saucers.

"I see," I said to the security guard. "What would you like me to do?"

"You go in there and get him to stop."

He was short and pudgy, wearing a heavily padded jacket, a helmet, and a baton hanging from his belt. Going in on my own did not strike me as a good plan. My entire training in subduing agitated people consisted of a friendly nurse in the ER once showing me that if a person was lying down and you leaned your whole weight on his or her shoulder, it was tough for even a larger person to get up. This was helpful information, but not applicable. And that was the sum total of my skills. I asked the guard what would happen if we could not fix this. They would call the police, who would come in force and do whatever it took to subdue the patient, and then we could inject and sedate him. I looked back down the hall at the man slamming the door. I borrowed the supervisor's white coat. Usually I disliked the trappings of authority, but in that moment, I clutched at any useful tool. The guard did not want to enter the unit, but eventually agreed to walk behind me. I didn't want to appear like the coward I was, so I pulled my 112 pounds and borrowed white coat into a costume of concerned dignity. This was the moment in my life when I was most frightened.

We walked down the endless corridor. I stopped a few feet from the patient, where he could see me well. The guard stopped quite a bit farther back. The man held the door and looked at me. I said, "The nurses are stuck in there and it's time for them to go home. I am hoping you'll go in your room. Then they can leave." He looked at me. He looked at the nurses in their glass bunker. He knew this drill infinitely better than I did—the police, the takedown, restraints, needles. He put his arm down and walked quietly into the room. The security guard instantly skipped forward, closing and locking the door.

So yes, sometimes one must consider restraints for a patient who is *furiously mad*. During the week I write this, a young doctor was punched in the face, hard, by a psychotic patient in an emergency room in New York City. More training and more staffing can help limit their use and abuse. Advocates of moral treatment made these same arguments, insisting that good treatment for the mentally ill could almost entirely avoid restraints. Over time, though, Kirkbride's gentle persuasion failed; restraints held fast.

But moral treatment did not disappear without a trace. We will find its descendants, when we look at today's best treatments for dementia. Back then, passionate advocates of reform were not content merely to write and speak about the benefits of compassion. They translated their idealism into concrete; they built mental hospitals across America. And it is there we will continue our search.

Chapter 3

The Big House: Its Rise and Fall

In 1843, firebrand reformer Dorothea Dix sent the Massachusetts legislature a paper to be read aloud on her behalf by a man, for women could neither vote nor speak to the legislature. Dix opens with a maidenly apology for the frank and unfeminine nature of her testimony. She then blasts her audience with tales of horror from across Massachusetts. Here is her report on the condition of one older woman, perhaps with dementia, and surely suffering like the damned:

> Late in December, 1842; thermometer 4° above zero; visited the almshouse . . . I asked to see the subject who was "out of doors;" and following the mistress of the house through the deep snow, shuddering and benumbed by the piercing cold, several hundred yards, we came in rear of the barn to a small building . . . in which was no fire, the rusty pipe seeming to threaten, in its decay, either suffocation by smoke, which by

and by we nearly realized, or conflagration of the building, together with destruction of its poor crazy inmate. . . . "Oh, I'm so cold, so cold," was uttered in plaintive tones by a woman within the cage; "oh, so cold, so cold!" And well might she be cold; the stout, hardy, driver of the sleigh had declared 'twas too hard for a man to stand the wind and snow that day, yet here was a woman caged and imprisoned without fire or clothes, not naked indeed, for one thin cotton garment partly covered her, and part of a blanket was gathered about the shoulders; there she stood, shivering in that dreary place, the grey locks falling in disorder about the face gave a wild expression to the pallid features; untended and comfortless, she might call aloud, none could hear; she might die, and there be none to close the eye. But death would have been a blessing here.[1]

Dix looked hard at sights others chose to ignore. She saw people who were not only poor but ill, and called for some response other than the poorhouse. A proper New Englander, Dix changed the way Americans cared for "insane paupers." By the time she died in 1887, a burgeoning system of mental hospitals was an increasingly common destination for the mentally ill, for Dix believed that a hospital was the place for compassionate care. As the mentally ill entered hospitals, so too did those with dementia, and that is where our search takes us now.

Dix's view—that the indigent mentally ill deserved kindness and treatment—was controversial, even radical. As we trace the history of responses toward the poor, cognitively impaired, and old, Dix's work offers an important flexion point: She directly attacked stigma against the mentally ill, and in so doing, changed the way Americans saw at least some of those who were poor. She undermined the notion that poverty is a choice by demonstrating that the mentally ill had no say in the matter. Dix crisscrossed the states, visiting the mentally ill where they were so she could see for herself the conditions in which they lived.

Dix's early years forged her soul into that of a reformer. She was born in 1802 to a chilly and remote family in Maine. In her infancy, her father took to the road as a preacher. Her mother, forty-two years old at Dorothea's birth, was an invalid and seems to have made miserable company. Dix declined to speak of those austere early years, except to say, "I never knew childhood."[2] She escaped by twelve to live in Boston with her grandmother, where she found material comfort and social standing, but no greater warmth.[3]

As a young woman, Dix joined her grandmother's circle of Boston luminaries, including Ralph Waldo Emerson and William Ellery Channing, the "father of Unitarianism," and set herself a demanding schedule of working and teaching. She battled tuberculosis throughout her life, along with bouts of crippling depression. In 1836, she left Boston for a restorative yearlong trip to Europe, where she met Samuel Tuke and was impressed by his views on care for the mentally ill. Upon her return, a newly fired-up Dix went to the East Cambridge jail to offer lessons in Scripture to incarcerated women. There she found mentally ill inmates kept in unheated cells and deplorable conditions. Dix was galvanized. She took up as her cause the humane treatment of the mentally ill. But political action for women in 1840 was no easy matter. She couldn't run for office. She couldn't vote. She could not even testify before the legislature.

Then as now, the vulnerable end up where others let them fall. Dix undertook, at her own expense, a survey of the indigent mentally ill in every "almshouse, workhouse and prison" in Massachusetts.[4] It took her eighteen months. A woman of her era and class was meant to live a sheltered life, shielded from every offensive sight, smell, and thought. Dix forced her way into scenes of filth and degradation, taking copious notes. She saw men and women naked, living in their own excrement; she listened to them curse in ways she had never imagined. She saw their chains and heard them howl. She held her testimony up as a mirror to the public of Massachusetts.

Dix and her contemporaries largely succeeded in their battle to hospitalize the mentally ill. She had a hand in building more than thirty mental hospitals in the United States. Many incorporated the tenets of moral treatment. When New York Hospital opened a psychiatric facility in 1821, advice from Dr. Tuke shaped its site and appearance. The Bloomingdale Insane Asylum was constructed in an elevated spot with "an extensive and delightful view of the Hudson, the East river, and the Bay and Harbour of New York."[5] One building still remains—Columbia University's Buell Hall, which once housed wealthy male inmates. Its elegant design was intended to avoid anything that might "impress [patients'] minds with the idea of a prison, or a place of punishment."[6] These new asylums were built at a distance from cities, so that residents might enjoy tranquil surroundings, pleasant vistas, and the opportunity to enjoy nature. The program generally focused on clear rules and structured activities, with early and regular hours.[7] Patients enjoyed simple healthy meals and light manual labor. Men worked on the farm, milking cows and growing vegetables, while women had lighter duties like basket weaving, all based on a faith in the healing power of simplicity, work, and the natural world.[8]

In these early decades of the nineteenth century, a buoyant optimism swept up experts concerned with mental illness. No longer need the mentally ill suffer in jails and prisons. They would be healed by the new moral treatment and the magnificent establishments that housed it. Or so claimed Horace Mann in 1832, in a report to the Massachusetts legislature pleading for funds for the unfinished Worcester Asylum. While Bloomingdale was a private establishment, Worcester would be a public facility sheltering impoverished patients. Even so, they would benefit from large windows and lofty ceilings, providing healing "light and pure air." A patient might have a private attendant to "remain constantly at his side, to occupy his attention with pleasing themes" and walk with him "into the open air, the fields and the woods, that the restorative influences of nature might strike some chord in the heart."[9] We will see Mann's arguments for better funding arise again and again. First, he says, it is the right thing to provide humane and scientific treatment, and set aside the whips and chains of the past. Second, government will *save money* by eradicating a terrible disease. Keeping the insane in jails, where they never recover, incurs enormous expense, whereas mental illness can be cured if treated early and skillfully. As Mann says, "Pecuniary interest, then becomes the auxiliary of duty."[10] His fiscal argument was the more persuasive, and is echoed by arguments today about the great savings to be won by curing dementia. (Alas, it didn't work for mental illness then, and will not work for dementia today.)

Ultimately, nineteenth-century psychiatric treatment failed to live up to this gilded win-win vision. The Worcester Asylum was built. Designed for 120 patients, it had expanded to hold 255 by the time of Dix's testimony to the legislature. By 1843, the trustees aimed for 400 beds. The expansions at Worcester only hinted at the building spree to come. Across the country, public mental institutions could not keep pace with demand; they grew in number, doubling between 1870 and 1890.[11] Hospitals supersized, packing 800 or 1,000 patients into facilities meant for 100. This growth depended on strong support from legislators, but as more and more money flowed toward mental hospitals, the politicians' whining grew louder. No one had known the need was so great. Who were all these patients?

More pertinent to our investigation: How many of these patients had dementia? It's hard to say. The Worcester census lists "dementia" as a common diagnosis, but their dementia is not ours. The director noted that these patients "often improve very soon, and almost always recover. They are extremely likely to forget all that passed while in this torpid state."[12] More likely this is what we would call delirium, a temporary clouding of consciousness.

In the 1880 census, people over the age of sixty-five made up only 3.4 percent of the overall population, yet they were 17 percent of the mental hospital population. Many of these older patients likely had dementia, though their presence is masked by changing definitions and diagnoses. Typical of those institutionalized was this older woman, as described by her son: "Of late she has grown materially worse, so that we deem it unsafe for the female portion of the family to be left alone with her during the day and especially unsafe for the little 2 year old that is obliged to remain continually there, as she has stated several times of late that she or the children must be sacrificed."[13]

Money and the support of a family made all the difference, then and now. Around that time, Ralph Waldo Emerson developed dementia, gradually losing his ability to write, remember, comprehend, and even speak beyond a few words. Revered by his family and wide circle of friends, Emerson was able to remain at home. His devoted daughter Ellen cared for him, traveled with him, and did her best to shield him from embarrassment. (The cost of care was understood differently then; his adult daughter was expected to care for him, and lacked other options for employment.) Emerson's extraordinary stature in American society meant he could continue giving public lectures, though these were less and less well received as his dementia advanced. Over time, he could no longer reliably read aloud his published works without confusion.[14]

Celebrated or not, older people with dementia merited little discussion in the medical journals of the day. There was, however, a group of patients who drew great interest. General paresis mattered, for it was a dementia predominantly of the young, not the old, and more common in men than women. Dozens of articles on general paresis pop up in the medical literature of the 1850s to 1890s. One report notes that it differs from "simple insanity, because paresis shows anatomical changes."[15] Nineteenth-century physicians could not find pathology in the brains of those with depression or mania, but here they saw diminished folds in the brain's cortex. Because of those lesions, general paresis fueled a vigorous debate, ranging over decades, about whether or not mental illnesses arise from objective changes in the brain.

Countless doctors took up the study. In 1863, a Swedish scholar walked colleagues through the phases of the illness, starting with abnormalities in gait and progressing to incontinence. Victims were predominantly men between the ages of twenty-five and forty, and doctors often found "vicious habits" of a sexual nature, likely coded language for sex between men; female patients were often prostitutes.[16] In the final, fatal stage, a patient is bed-bound and mute; such a "man dies while still alive, for it is only the animal which breathes and assimilates . . . The patient is only a burden, a mass of foetid lumber here upon earth."[17] In the 1870s, when overcrowded mental institutions were a matter of growing concern, more than 10 percent of inpatients were diagnosed with general paresis.[18] By the end of the century, some doctors estimated nearly half of institutionalized patients had the disease.[19]

In 1877, Dr. Alexander E. Macdonald, superintendent of the New York City Asylum for the Insane, presented his scientific observations on general paresis.[20] Dr. Macdonald had carefully studied the pattern of dissemination in the population. It started in one locality with men, spread gradually in men, and then appeared in women. By the 1870s, the disease had spread from the East Coast to areas in the South and West. Incredibly, Dr. Macdonald, capable of providing such accurate observations of the pattern of spread, could not in that era recognize that such a disease was infectious, and more specifically a sexually transmitted infectious disease. It was, he argued, hereditary—that would explain the inclusion of prostitutes, since they were corrupt from the start. The debate raged on for the rest of the century, until scientific advances like the Wassermann test and the identification of the treponeme, the bacterium that causes syphilis, won the day. Denial gradually gave way to a rueful admission that almost all cases of general paresis resulted from late-stage syphilis.

Why should psychiatrists have so strongly resisted the connection? Right from the start there were strong indications of a link. Only willful blindness prevented the field from accepting it. Many psychiatrists were pleased to find a disease that had mental symptoms and brain pathology—proof, they thought, that such a link must always exist. More important, perhaps general paresis, unlike chronic mental illnesses, might be cured. Instead of filling mental hospitals with old, incurable patients, psychiatrists hoped to provide dramatic lifesaving help to young ones. Both pride and money were on the line. Many communities had raised the mentally ill out of almshouses and jails and into stately mental hospitals, but questions remained about whether the "indigent insane" really deserved large public expenditures. A connection between mental illness and vice could be ruinous. It would be better for psychiatry, and for the public view of the mentally ill, if the link was ignored.

The battle over general paresis was part of a larger war for American psychiatry. More and more patients were hospitalized for decades, and these long-stay cases were filling up the hospitals. Psychiatrists and reformers had promised that treatment quickly provided at the start of illness would cure the mentally ill, but it was clear they could not deliver. By 1882, they could not deny the huge expense of these institutions and the frustrating continued need for more beds. One exasperated superintendent puts the blame on those whose "insanity is associated with crime, with drunkenness, with epilepsy, with congenital defects."[21] If only the hospitals could rid themselves of undesirable patients, there would be enough room for those who might be cured.

The number of people who were old, poor, and showing signs of dementia steadily increased. Almshouses were generally funded by counties and local communities, and mental institutions by the state. Suddenly, local governments strapped for funds discovered that these people were not primarily impoverished; instead, they suffered mainly from mental illness, so off they went to the state-funded mental institution. No doubt officials were partly inspired by the message of mercy from reformers like Kirkbride and Dix, but they also couldn't help but notice that local finances improved when this population moved to the state-funded mental hospital. This was the first time, but far from the last, that a shift in funding led to a change of diagnosis and of domicile for the vulnerable.[22]

The shift from almshouses to public mental hospitals was accelerated by such laws as the New York State Care Act in 1890. The bill required county institutions to transfer those with mental illness to state hospitals as soon as possible. These larger institutions, legislators hoped, would provide care that was more economical, more consistent, and more readily supervised.[23] Similar reforms in Massachusetts and other states vastly increased the number of people in state institutions.

Laws like these were not aimed at people with dementia. Nonetheless, demented elders profoundly felt their impact for the next fifty years. From roughly 1890 until after World War II, the population of state mental institutions mushroomed, especially the population of elders. In Massachusetts, the number of men older than sixty at first admission quadrupled, while rates of admission for other age groups stayed roughly the same. This change is striking. Only rarely do major mental illnesses arise in older age—schizophrenia and bipolar illness are far more likely to emerge in one's twenties. The major exception to this rule is dementia, which is the disease most likely to first emerge at age sixty or older. Other states racked up similar demographic changes. In New York, by the middle of the twentieth century, fully 40 percent of patients first admitted to mental hospitals were older than sixty.[24] At the peak in 1955, well over 500,000 Americans lived in state facilities.

The movement to build state mental hospitals started with the zeal of reformers like Dorothea Dix. Nothing gold can stay; the reformers' idealized vision decayed into a distinctly more troubling reality. The well-funded, well-staffed, and restraint-free hospital of Dr. Kirkbride gradually faded. By 1900, state institutions were as overcrowded as the jails and poorhouses had been in centuries past and lacked the lofty goals and innovative programs of earlier years—no more milking cows and weaving baskets. The limited, poorly trained staff did not calm the agitated with the gentle suasion of moral treatment. Bedstraps and straitjackets forced unruly patients to toe the line.[25] But though they did not cure mental illness, mental hospitals survived, for they had carved out a useful niche, that of containing those unable to care for themselves and without families willing and able to care for them.

It is alluring to imagine a time when family and community cared lovingly for frail older relatives. But the care of sick elders has long fallen to government. And for just as long, governments have grumbled about the cost of that care. America has long strained between two responses. One is pragmatic to the point of cruelty and seeks the cheapest, easiest means to keep discarded people out of the way. Punishment, starvation, shame—all are acceptable as long as costs are low. The second response overflows with idealism, striving to heal or at least comfort the needy. Moral treatment raised up the art of caring as an important aspect of treatment for mental illness. It also had a solid basis in clinical observations, by showing that people thrived in an environment of respect. It attempted to unite a scientific, modern, manly approach to medicine with the compassion and care that are often enough viewed as womanly, the province of nurses. The legacy of choosing cure over care haunts us today, when a cure still eludes those with dementia, and the need for care grows ever greater.

Mental hospitals built to the specifications of Thomas Kirkbride still mark the American landscape, in Ohio and Georgia and upstate New York. These ghostly buildings are shuttered and rapidly deteriorating, glass panes shattered in the many large windows. Moral treatment, made concrete by these buildings, came under fire in subsequent generations. Healthy food, respectful care, and comfortable surroundings did not cure mental illness; the rate of serious illness continued on without change. The critics were right. Kindness cannot cure mental illness, any more than it can cure cancer or cardiac disease. Compassion, respect, food, and physical liberty are not a cure. They are only the necessary conditions for any human flourishing. And without that humane context, no treatment can work. In rejecting moral treatment, later generations failed to preserve the best of the old ways, and left Dr. Kirkbride's spirit to rot along with his buildings.

Chapter 4

Exitus Letalis

J ust at the turn from the nineteenth century to the twentieth, dementia steps out of the shadows and into the light—but only for a moment. Dementia was always there, hiding in plain sight, but now at last it falls within the gaze of scientists. And then dementia returns to the shadows, waiting for another moment of recognition.

It is not as if dementia was impossible to see. Families cared for aging relatives whose cognitive function faded, sometimes slowly and steadily, sometimes fast and drastically. They did the best they could, while physicians and scientists paid essentially no attention—dementia in the elderly was not a topic of research. Instead, it was just a part of aging—irreversible, untreatable, and uninteresting. Then something started to change. There were more old people, and more old people with dementia. Those people sometimes lacked families, and even those with families could be hard to care for at home. By the start of the twentieth century, more and more elders with dementia had entered the vast system of mental institutions. They rarely left, except in death.

The *American Journal of Insanity* (*AJI*), the premier journal on mental illness of the day, is a rough guide for measuring research interest in dementia. (The title was formally changed in July 1921 to the *American Journal of Psychiatry*, and remains a premier source of psychiatric research.) If we look carefully, there are no articles on the topic from the journal's founding in 1844 until 1897, when a brief case study appears.[1] A few years later, in 1902, William Russell of the Willard State Hospital in New York publishes the first full article in the *American Journal of Insanity* on dementia in the elderly.[2] Russell explicitly worries about elders filling up the hospital where he works. For the prior decade a quarter of admissions had been patients over sixty. He tries to parse out the difference between normal cognitive aging and dementia. Old demented people get admitted to the asylum and stay a long time, causing him problems. He's not happy about it.

Russell's paper is the first among many that focus, with increasing anxiety, on the problem of institutionalized elders with dementia. Once the Great Depression hits, the murmurs turn into a roar as loud as a biplane. Richard Hutchings, in his 1939 president's address to the American Psychiatric Association, laments the fivefold increase in elders with dementia then in New York state mental institutions. Communities who "pass on the burden and expense of the aged and unwanted . . . threaten to convert state hospitals into vast infirmaries for dotards."[3]

The daunting numbers of elderly patients in mental hospitals spark the first faint glimmerings of scientific interest in dementia.

I n 1903, Alois Alzheimer sought associates to work in his lab in Munich. This post was among the most prestigious in the world for a physician-scientist seeking training. Alzheimer selected five interns that year. Only one was American. He was also African American.

How did this young man, Solomon Carter Fuller, get to Germany? And what did he do with his knowledge when he came back to the United States?

Fuller took a circuitous route to Alzheimer's cutting-edge lab. His paternal grandparents were American slaves who bought their freedom, left Virginia, and emigrated to Liberia in 1852, joining the movement of free blacks to create a nation there. Their son established a coffee plantation in Liberia, where Solomon was born in 1872. His maternal grandparents were medical missionaries, and from them, Fuller gleaned an interest in medicine. By the time Fuller was a teenager, America was no longer the country his grandparents had left. Slavery, if not its legacy, was a thing of the past.

And so it was that at seventeen years old, Solomon Fuller sailed for America, seeking an education. He landed in North Carolina and graduated four years later from Livingstone College, a historically black institution in its early years. He then studied at Long Island College Hospital Medical School and later at Boston University, graduating with his medical degree in 1897.[4] Fuller landed an internship for two years at the Westborough State Hospital for the Insane. Fuller's interest was not only in psychiatry but in brain pathology, yet the value of pathologists to psychiatry was not universally accepted. The search for correlations between brain abnormalities and mental illness was just getting started, and many were skeptical that such links existed—and continued to be so for generations to come. Fuller's abundant intellectual curiosity and ambition led him to take up the work of autopsies on patients who died at Westborough. This was a task shunned by others, but Fuller gained knowledge and experience that set him ahead of his peers. His genius was for the careful, correct observation of phenomena that others didn't bother to inspect. He created value and opportunity from a position that others dismissed.

Having arrived as a teenage African immigrant, he secured an education, a job, and superior training.

When he completed his internship, Fuller was appointed pathologist at Westborough; this job brought along an academic appointment as instructor in pathology at Boston University Medical College. For the next three years, he perfected his techniques, making slides of his autopsy studies and recording clinical case histories. But Fuller was not yet content with his training.

He contacted the celebrated pathologist Edward K. Dunham and moved to Bellevue in New York, where he honed his skills by performing autopsies in their vast morgue. Dunham was impressed with Fuller's work, and counseled him that the very best American physicians, including Dunham himself, had studied in Europe. The opportunities for scientific study in the United States just could not compare with those in the academic centers of Germany, England, and France. If European study was what the best did, Fuller would do this, too. He applied for the highly competitive position in Alzheimer's lab and got the job.

Alzheimer's connections read like a who's who of German science. He made his mark by mastering the cell-staining techniques pioneered by his supervisor, Dr. Franz Nissl, at Frankfurt's Municipality Asylum for the Mentally Sick and Epileptics.[5] Alzheimer's mentor, Emil Kraepelin, was one of the great minds in psychiatry and the author of the standard text in the field. Alzheimer displayed many of the features of today's clinician researchers, working with patients to understand clinical symptoms and then trying to ferret out links between those symptoms and specific pathology in the brain.

Fuller worked with Alzheimer in Munich from 1903 to 1905. German was the language of science and Alzheimer's lab, so Fuller worked in German, learning the newest and most advanced techniques then available for examining brain tissue. He absorbed an intellectual atmosphere of extraordinary richness. With Alzheimer as his mentor, Fuller worked at the epicenter of science. In 1905, Fuller came home to Westborough as one of a handful of elite European-educated physicians, with skills and knowledge in brain pathology to rival the best American scholars of the day. True to the ethos of Alzheimer, Fuller continued his work in pathology and also established a practice in clinical psychiatry, the better to study correlations between brain lesions and symptoms.

Fuller debuts in the world of scientific publication in April 1907. Let's take a trek through what he brought to the science of dementia. For me, it's worth the trip. Fuller starts with an exhaustive study on neurofibrils, a type of tiny strand found in nerve cells.[6] Fuller's paper is a knockout—a technical tour de force that differs radically from most articles in the decades before and after. His standards for scientific evidence and reasoning are impeccable—unlike many publications of the day. He is more comprehensive as well. Most publications in the *American Journal of Insanity* at that time are fewer than ten pages long. Fuller's tome is sixty-seven pages, including plate after plate of exquisite drawings and photographs of his microscopic studies of brain cells. It's essentially a dissertation, taking the up-to-the-minute techniques Fuller perfected in Alzheimer's lab and applying them to the study of patients in the Westborough Asylum. Fuller reviews in detail the relevant literature on neurofibrils—for the prior seventy years, since the first report of their discovery in 1838.[7] He is particularly concerned with the degeneration of neurofibrils, describing in detail their "fragmentation, adhesion, and swelling" in the brains of the patients he has examined. He offers a wealth of clinical case detail, reporting the puzzling behavior of one older Harvard graduate who exercised by "running on the streets in abbreviated costume." He specifically addresses the sort of neurofibril changes associated with different diseases of the brain, including senile dementia, finally known by a name recognizable to us, and advanced syphilis. He gets right to the brink of work that will shortly thereafter make Alzheimer famous, though he doesn't draw Alzheimer's conclusions. The paper is a sequoia among seedlings. It reveals the work of a beautiful mind, patiently applying the best laboratory science of the day to the puzzle of clinical symptoms in different illnesses, including dementia. His thoroughness, his pursuit of objective evidence, and his discipline in assessing what the data do and do not demonstrate show a command of the scientific method unsurpassed by other researchers of the day.

However, it was a different paper on neurofibrils, one by Alzheimer, that went on to become famous. A few years before Fuller's time in Germany, in November 1901, Alzheimer examined a patient known in the annals of medical history as Auguste D. The published description of her illness, along with a small number of other cases, comprise the earliest reports of what came to be known as Alzheimer's disease. Auguste D was fifty-one when admitted to the hospital; she had been happily married with one child. She had been healthy until March of 1901, when she accused her husband of strolling inappropriately about with a female neighbor. Next, memory lapses began. Two months later she "started making mistakes in preparing meals, paced nervously and without reason in the apartment, and was not careful with the household money."[8] Auguste D became frightened of local tradespeople and of dying. By November, she could no longer recall her address or her husband's name; she could not write her own name. Her condition went from bad to worse. She became bed-bound and developed a bedsore, which became infected, which caused pneumonia. Auguste D died of these complications of dementia in 1906.

By that time Alzheimer no longer worked in Frankfurt. He asked that her record and brain be sent to him in Munich for examination. He presented her case at a psychiatric conference in 1906 and published his account in a psychiatric journal in 1907.[9] Alzheimer described the "tangled bundles of fibers" that had taken over some of her neurons, as well as deposits dispersed throughout her cortex. Alzheimer used the most advanced techniques available in his day. He wasn't the first to describe plaques and neurofibrils, but he linked tangled neurofibrils to the disease that now bears his name. These plaques and tangles form a core of current basic science research on dementia.

What made Auguste D's case interesting was precisely that she was not old. Her early onset dementia, coupled with those odd neuropathological findings, became known as Alzheimer's disease. Alzheimer didn't name the disease of early onset dementia for himself. Kraepelin, his mentor, designated the syndrome as a new disease in his 1910 textbook, though only a few such cases had been observed at the time.[10]

Alzheimer's work did not go unnoticed in America. Studies of brain pathology in dementia and other diseases started to appear in medical publications. In 1908, C. M. Campbell cited Alzheimer as he tried to distinguish between dementia caused by old age from dementia caused by changes in blood vessels.[11] A few years later, E. E. Southard's 1910 paper on the anatomy of senile dementia offers strong clinical observations and common sense that fairly leap from the page.[12] He had worked with a young Harvard medical student, a "Mr. N. S. Burns," to prepare case histories and matching pathology for twenty-three cases of senile dementia. Southard makes an insightful observation: He can't see why patients with dementia must stay in the asylum. Many are weak, blind, and deaf, but surely these problems could be handled, perhaps better, elsewhere.

Back in the United States, Fuller continued his research on

dementia as well; his papers stand out for the clear thinking and honest scholarship that were his hallmark. (More interesting still, Fuller reached conclusions that were controversial in his day and yet were validated by scholarship decades later.) They require real effort to parse, being more like small dense books than like typical articles of the time. Yet they also engage the reader. Typically they weave together Latin terms, medical data, and poignant snatches of conversation between doctor and patient. For example: "Q: Where is your home? A: I have no home but hopple popple home all the time." Many of these case summaries end with ultimate finality: *Exitus letalis*, or the lethal outcome.[13] Then as now, dementia kills.

In one paper, coauthored with colleague Henry Klopp, Fuller questions whether Alzheimer's disease deserves to be viewed as a distinct entity, defined as a syndrome with all the clinical and pathological features of dementia in older people, but occurring in younger patients.[14] Among American physicians, Fuller was uniquely positioned to understand and evaluate Alzheimer's work—and he had reservations. Fuller presents a case of a woman dying of dementia in her fifties. Her brain shows no tangled neurofibrils—none at all. She has plaques, but these are neither large nor numerous. (Based on the case description, this patient might today meet criteria for frontotemporal dementia.) He doesn't find any distinctive pathology in other young patients with dementia. He asks, "What are we to understand by senility in an anatomical or psychiatric sense? Anatomically we are as yet unable to draw a line with a degree of precision between the brain of some so-called normal elderly persons and certain senile dements."[15] He specifically hesitates to "reduce senile dementia to terms of plaques." Fuller, speaking clearly but courteously to his old mentor, finds there is insufficient justification to name a disease based on early onset dementia after Alzheimer. His conclusion: There are insufficient differences in pathology to justify separating dementia in the young from dementia in the old.

Fuller was prescient. Though his observations were largely forgotten, in the 1970s neuroscientists finally agreed that there are not two forms of dementia merely separated by age.[16] Sixty years after Fuller's research, the category of Alzheimer's disease was enlarged to include dementia in people exhibiting pathological plaques and tangles, whether young or old.

Fuller also produced a paper that investigated the role of "miliary plaques" in the brains of the elderly, noting that there had been insufficient work on dementia, "largely for the reason of a commonly expected fatal outcome in a mental disease affecting persons already near the end of the allotted span of life."[17] To fill in those gaps in the scientific record, Fuller offers an exhaustive review of what was known to date about plaques in the brain. He provides supporting arguments for his point of view as carefully as an engineer calculates support for a bridge. He constructs a study precisely to assess the relationships between plaques, dementia, and old age. He compares the brains of thirty-three elderly patients dying "insane" to those of fifty young patients who died with mental illness and six elderly patients who died without mental illness. He serves up a wealth of clinical detail so that the reader may assess the evidence for his conclusions. He describes, for instance, a man in good health until age eighty-three, who then lost his memory, took to wandering from his home in an "aimless and confused manner," and "on one occasion very nearly killed his aged wife by choking her." He describes another "man of 80 years of age and without psychosis who exhibited plaques in abundance."[18] He cites the work of other scholars who found plaques in the brains of only half of elderly patients dying with the symptoms of dementia and concludes that plaques are not caused by arteriosclerosis, contrary to the common belief of the day. He argues that though plaques are commonly found in the brains of those with senile dementia, they "cannot be considered as characteristic for any special form of mental disease." Plaques were found in the brains of older persons without mental illness and in the brains of young persons with many illnesses, including syphilis.[19] Some people whose symptoms matched senile dementia had none. He concludes that pathological differences between the brain in senile dementia and in old age are more of degree than kind.

Astonishingly, Fuller finds that plaques are neither necessary nor sufficient for dementia in the elderly. I have to pause here for a moment to catch my breath. Fuller's conclusion, ignored for roughly a hundred years, is the destination at which many—though by no means all—neuropathologists have arrived today, after decades of acrimonious debate. Consider the Nun Study, an impressive long-term project that generated publications starting around 2000 that cover years of research. In it, we'll find confirmation that Alzheimer-like plaques and tangles do not always correlate with symptoms of dementia.[20] Again, in 2014, major clinical trials fail, leading to the discovery that a third of the expert-referred patients with supposed Alzheimer's dementia had insufficient plaques to merit the diagnosis.[21] Fuller could have predicted—in fact, actually *did* predict—the outcome of these major studies, but the brilliant scientists who study dementia had undergone their own collective memory loss.

It's hard to know precisely why Fuller didn't receive more recognition during his lifetime or since. Certainly racism played a big role. Contemporaries with his level of expertise went on to leadership positions not open to him; they enjoyed far more opportunities to present their work and theories to the scientific community. But perhaps Fuller was also at a disadvantage because of the inconvenient nature of his skepticism. If his findings had coincided with those of a new generation of researchers, if he had argued in favor of a linear relationship between plaques, tangles, and dementia, perhaps he would have been more celebrated. Had we held on to Fuller's observations, there might have been less puzzlement at current work that questions the links that Fuller similarly questioned. Had Fuller's work received the attention it deserved, both initially and in subsequent generations, maybe we'd be further along today in understanding and treating dementia.

The flurry of interest in dementia lasted for roughly ten years. And then, for the most part, that interest died; this line of research recedes into obscurity for decades. There are a small number of studies, but these excite little notice. Psychiatrists for the most part drop the study of brain anatomy altogether. By 1928, Adolf Meyer, in his presidential address to the American Psychiatric Association, ridicules his own early work in pathology as a time "when real science in medicine was identified with the deadhouse and the use of the microscope."[22] The scientific study of dementia would not revive until the 1970s, enough time for a child to be born during Fuller's era, live and grow old, and develop dementia.

Solomon Fuller did not live to see the resurgence of scientific interest in dementia. His work was acknowledged in his own time by the small circle of researchers able to appreciate it. On the strength of his research and his connections with prestigious European researchers, he was invited to attend Freud's celebrated visit to lecture at Clark University in 1909; he can barely be seen in the last spot in the last row of the classic photo from this occasion. He deserves more of a spotlight in the history of neuroscience.

If he did not receive the professional recognition he deserved,

Fuller's home life had its joys. In 1906 he met the artist Meta Warrick, a sculptor and poet who became a celebrated figure in the Harlem Renaissance. Fuller wooed her with such a splendid dinner that Meta preserved the menu all her life, with its Lobster Newberg, wine, pink and green ribbons, flowers, and ferns.[23] They married in 1909, and lived in Framingham, Massachusetts. Though neighbors tried to prevent them from moving into the fine house that Fuller had built, they lived there for decades, raising three sons.[24] His affectionate letters include one addressed to her as "Dear Little Sweetheart," that sends "all the love of my heart to you and the children."[25] He was a devoted gardener, earning this description from a white neighbor in the 1930s: "His beautiful flower garden is the one recreation of the most interesting person in our town. Slight of stature, quiet, unassuming, kindly, a keen judge of human nature, a gentleman in every respect is our colored physician."[26]

Fuller left Westborough State Hospital in 1919, after nearly twenty years, and moved to Boston University, where he was the sole African American on the faculty. He was paid a small stipend to teach pathology, yet shamefully, he was never formally placed on the payroll.[27] He consulted for other facilities, including the Veterans Hospital in Tuskegee, Alabama, for which he helped train several African American psychiatrists. He served five years as chair of the department of neurology at Boston University, though again he was slighted—he was welcome to do the work but never officially received the title of chair. He resigned from the faculty when a young white physician was made chair in his place.

In science and in life, Fuller the clear-eyed pathologist knew how to look, and he knew what he saw, whether it was neuropathology or

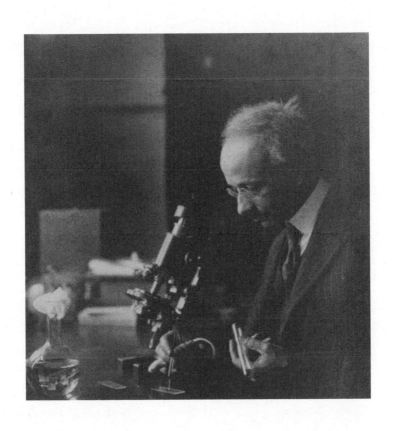

racism. He was a quiet revolutionary. He did his work and did it remarkably well. He appreciated recognition, but did not appear to expect it. Even in a system set up to drown out his views and his standing, he drew his own conclusions. As we look back, a hundred years later, we see it all so easily. Fuller's vision was wonderfully clear. If only we had paid more attention.

Chapter 5

Darkness into Light

I n the 1970s, politics, money, and science all weave together to bring dementia—as a political problem, a clinical entity, and a topic of research—out of the shadows. How did this transition from darkness into light happen?

To understand the evolution, we'll examine the first half of the twentieth century, a time of many discoveries in medicine, but simultaneously a dark era. These were the years in which medicine set aside the ancient principle: First, do no harm. Physician-scientists grew bold, unleashing radical experimental treatments. Serious illnesses in all domains of medicine were attacked by powerful methods. Radical cancer surgeries, chemotherapies, and a host of aggressive interventions shaped the new war on disease.[1] The war metaphor is quite apt; for example, the battle against breast cancer left many women scarred, not always with benefit to their health.[2] Some experimental efforts led to successful treatments; most did not. We can now treat more illnesses, and those are important gains. But the injuries and loss of life were high. Patients died of these experiments, some suffering terribly. Physicians called invasive experimental treatments heroic, but who is the hero here? The doctors were like generals, high up on their horses, surveying the field from a promontory. It was the patients, like foot soldiers, who made the ultimate sacrifice. Physicians thought the risk worth the possible gain; what patients thought is unclear. Standards for gaining consent were rudimentary, as were requirements that treatments demonstrate safety and efficacy before their use in human beings.

Psychiatrists were frustrated by crowded hospitals and the lack of effective treatments for severe mental illness. Aggressive methods were taken up for clearing out the asylum. Racism and nativism gathered steam; immigrants and minorities were singled out as vectors of mental illness. One typical article finds a high frequency among "Hebrews" of psychosis, and a paucity of anxiety in the "happy go lucky Negroes."[3] And why would that be? Heredity was the issue! What better way to stop mental illness than by preventing mentally ill people from having children? The presidential address of 1908 to the American Medico-Psychological Association urges society to "prevent the marriage of the feeble-minded."[4] Between 1900 and 1950, sterilization programs emerged as a major weapon in the campaign against mental illness. States across the country enacted laws permitting the sterilization of "mental defectives"—California and Virginia were especially active. Though thousands of such operations were permitted over patients' objections, some physicians called for more, for "this protection has not been given to a large proportion of those by whom it is needed."[5]

Sterilization could wipe out future generations of "defectives," but could not weed out older patients in asylums. What to do? Some localities took to sending "quiet dements" out to board with willing families in the community. (Those who favor "boarding out" always cite the Belgian village of Geel as a sterling example, even today. In its long history Geel has sometimes also served as an example of abuse.[6]) Some families successfully integrated the older person into their lives, forming warm relationships. Others showed more interest in the modest stipend, and frail elders went without adequate food, clothing, and shelter, much as they had when Dorothea Dix decried the shameful treatment of the mentally ill.

After the early decade of work by Alzheimer, Fuller, and others, there was little research in dementia, but psychiatry investigated other illnesses with enthusiasm. Many psychiatrists mocked the efforts of earlier scholars like Dr. Kirkbride, who promoted moral treatment and protected patients from beatings, chains, and starvation, and instead offered compassion and respect. True, moral treatment did not provide cures for dementia, mania, or psychosis. But it did keep those who suffered from mental illness out of harm's way.

The same cannot be said for the new scientific approach. From the 1920s through the 1960s, psychiatric patients faced invasive experimental treatments, generally without the right to refuse. Julius Wagner-Jauregg, who went on to win the Nobel Prize in 1927, observed that a patient with general paresis got briefly better after a bout of high fever.[7] Wagner-Jauregg set about intentionally exposing mental patients to infections in search of his "fever cure." He dabbled with the potentially lethal bugs that cause strep throat and tuberculosis, and then settled on malaria. A whopping 15 percent of patients died from his treatment, but psychotic symptoms disappeared, at least for a time, in some patients along the way. This era was a low-water mark in the cure/care continuum. Physicians literally got away with murder.

A patient might undergo insulin coma, as was done with John Forbes Nash Jr., the Princeton mathematician of *A Beautiful Mind*.[8] The most permanent of these interventions was lobotomy. The removal of brain tissue from the frontal lobes of patients not only limited agitation but rendered patients incapable of initiating much action at all. Hospital superintendents were pleased that staff need no longer deal with agitated patients; this was more of a permanent sedation than a cure. Since agitation was a key reason for a person to be confined, the lobotomy patient could be returned to the community, no longer living at the expense of the state, or so it was argued.

Lobotomy grew steadily in popularity through the 1930s until peaking in 1949, with more than 5,000 performed that year on U.S. mental patients. By 1951, physicians at more than half the mental institutions in the United States did lobotomies, and more than 18,000 people had undergone the procedure. Egas Moniz, the Portuguese physician who popularized lobotomy, won the Nobel Prize in 1949 for his work.[9] Within a few years, though, enthusiasm for the practice distinctly waned, as reports of complications and terrible side effects emerged.[10] For thousands of patients, the news arrived too late.

One treatment from this period still in use today is electroconvulsive therapy (ECT), known colloquially as shock treatment. In early years ECT was commonly associated with broken limbs, substantial memory loss, and other significant deleterious effects. Today's treatment is safe and effective, especially for depression, and uses low doses of energy, appropriate sedation, and careful selection of patients. ECT is easily dramatized and shows up in many fictional settings. For good or ill, these atmospheric portrayals shape public reactions to ECT far more than any scientific study.

Ironically, the presumption that elders with dementia would not respond to treatment had a protective effect. Leaders in the field like Karl and William Menninger promoted the message that "psychiatry has devoted itself in the past too much to the care of a hopeless and hapless few."[11] Scientists who wanted to cure mental illness rarely studied frail older patients, who had little chance of recovery—they would only mess up the research data—so most patients subjected to invasive treatment innovations were young. Relatively small numbers of patients with dementia underwent lobotomy. For the most part, they remained in the mental hospital, where their growing numbers made psychiatry and the governments who paid for their care see them as a burden, a problem to be solved.

Biological treatments weren't the only ones on the increase. The influence of Freud and psychoanalytic thought within psychiatry during the period can scarcely be overstated. More and more practitioners took on the analytic perspective, and prestigious posts and opportunities went to those allied with the psychodynamic approach.

These years revealed strains that had long been part of psychiatry. There were researchers and clinicians who focused on biological causes and treatments—for instance, by using lobotomy or insulin shock. Psychoanalysts took a different approach, hoping to revise the brain's structure through the universal cure, talking therapy. Each camp had important insights to offer. Each was capable of great error. Today there is no substantive dispute that biology plays a role in mental illness, as it does in all illness. Genes clearly influence the risk of developing schizophrenia and manic depression. At the same time, individual experiences and the environment also make an enormous difference, either positively or negatively. Medications can diminish many symptoms, and so can psychotherapy and cognitive treatment. Poverty and a lack of health care, good food, a solid education, and safe places to live, work, and play increase the risk for most forms of illness. Today we call these the social determinants of health, and a wealth of evidence supports the impact of these factors on health issues from heart disease to asthma to dementia.

Psychiatry built its empire on the mental hospital. These imposing edifices embodied psychiatry's lofty mission: to care for the mentally ill in a modern, competent way, and prevent the torments of jails and almshouses. Psychiatry's prestige and security grew from the mental asylum, for these institutions brought funding and a steady stream of jobs. But slowly, over time, the asylum ceased to be a fortress for psychiatry and became instead a prison. The twentieth century saw a steady drumbeat of scandals involving mental institutions, reaching a crescendo after World War II. Limited funding, decaying physical plants, and falling ratios of staff to patients made for deteriorating conditions in state hospitals. Not only was the population of mental institutions surprisingly large, it was old. And not only were these patients old, they were demented. In 1946, 43.7 percent of first admissions were for organic brain syndrome, a diagnosis that closely matches today's diagnosis of dementia.[12]

By the end of the 1940s, calls for the reform of mental hospitals were widely broadcast. In 1946, Congress passed the National Mental Health Act, the first federal legislation to tackle psychiatric illness. This act created the National Institute of Mental Health (NIMH), which serves today as the primary section within the National Institutes of Health (NIH) for funding research on psychiatric illnesses. Robert Felix, the founding director of NIMH, was installed in 1949. One of his earliest and most significant battles was to have NIMH included with the other institutes as part of NIH, as the original legislation did not locate mental illness within NIH and thus within the rest of medicine.

Every generation sees with remarkable clarity the mistakes of the generation before. Innovators come up with new and better solutions to intractable problems, or so they believe until another generation comes along, shaking their heads in dismay. So it has been with the question of what to do with people who are old, demented, and impoverished. As America grew and prospered in the twentieth century, the number of elders increased, and tens of thousands found their way to state-funded mental institutions.

Enter a new generation of reformers. The flaws of mental hospitals loomed large in a series of widely circulated exposés. By the 1950s, half a million people, including many with dementia, were institutionalized— a form of mass incarceration. That heralded panacea, the mental hospital, was no longer a solution. It was a disaster. It had to end immediately. Scandalous reports, coming fast one after another, documented just how unlikely the mental institution was to comfort patients, let alone cure them. *Life* magazine published Albert Maisel's exposé, "Bedlam, 1946," with photographs documenting conditions eerily like those in Europe's concentration camps.[13] That patients were used for hard labor, restrained, or left naked shocked readers across the country. Mary Jane Ward published her bestselling novel, *The Snake Pit*, further making vivid for the public the horrors of life in a mental institution.[14] The very same political entities that swept hundreds of thousands of people into these institutions were shocked, shocked to find them there.

Psychiatry was at a crossroads. Attempts to cure mental illness focused on either biologic or psychodynamic factors, though rarely both. Very little research addressed dementia in the elderly, even while these patients increasingly filled mental institutions. All those thousands of elders crowding the wards were nothing but "hopeless and hapless" cases, as psychiatrist Karl Menninger had decreed.[15] By 1961, a federal commission decreed that no new mental hospitals should be built. The thing now would be to get patients *out* of hospitals. An eerie swing of the pendulum, this recommendation mirrored legislation from the 1890s decreeing that the mentally ill must get out of poorhouses and *into* mental hospitals.

Psychiatrists had always resisted the view that mental illness was incurable, and that their work amounted only to custodial care for the mentally ill.[16] Now they pushed back with vigor. But no one imagined that frail elders with dementia could be cured. To make room for more promising patients, older people with chronic, unremitting disabilities should go elsewhere. Directors of mental hospitals had been bellyaching for decades about having to care for all the wrong sorts of patients. Now they found a successful mechanism for shifting the care of elders somewhere else.

And what solution did the new generation discover? By the 1960s, the nursing home was the best place for those who were poor, old, alone, and demented. Cognitive decline and its symptoms no longer required mental health expertise; no treatment could cure the demented elder, so none need be offered. Custodial care was what they needed. In 1965, the creation of Medicare and Medicaid provided new funds to care for the elderly and the poor. New money added up to a new diagnosis and a new home.

The nursing home was not the worst place that elders with dementia could land. Through the 1960s and 1970s, many wound up on the streets, as part of the crisis of homelessness spawned by deinstitutionalization. The road to deinstitutionalization was paved with good intentions. Lots of people agreed that the half million patients in mental hospitals should no longer stay there. Advocates seized hold of the spirit of the 1960s and championed new rights for patients, drawing on the civil rights movements for minorities and women. State governments were increasingly concerned about the high cost of institutional care and saw community-based treatment as a way to save money. Psychiatrists celebrated successes in treating psychosis with drugs like chlorpromazine. All of these groups believed it was not only possible but necessary to free chronically hospitalized mental patients from institutions.

But the reality of deinstitutionalization was devastating. Hundreds of thousands of mental patients left institutions for America's neighborhoods. Some of those people had lived in hospitals for decades. Many were old. They had no job skills and little education. They had no money. They had lost track of or been abandoned by their families years ago. They suffered from illnesses like schizophrenia and manic depression and didn't know where they could now get treatment. They ended up living on the street in the full grip of severe mental illness.

Many patients could have safely lived in the community—if they had received proper support and treatment. But a robust network of community mental health centers, crucial for providing care to chronically ill people, simply never appeared. Housing support, job training, and all the programs that might have made transition possible were too few and too poorly funded.

The movement for deinstitutionalization succeeded in emptying mental institutions, but it failed to support lives of dignity and safety for those discharged. There can be no autonomy in the face of poverty and severe, untreated mental illness—unless a free fall without a safety net counts as liberty.[17] Once patients were no longer in state hospitals, they were, for many politicians, out of sight and out of mind.

Still, frail elders created a political problem for fans of deinstitutionalization. It was one thing to send psychotic but ambulatory adults to live on the street—one could pretend they just preferred homelessness. Who were we to limit their freedom? But how exactly would one discharge an older person who could not walk, speak, or feed herself? That would look really bad. The official responsible for sending grandma to live on a park bench would look very bad indeed. Instead of kicking everyone to the curb, some would be kicked into nursing homes.

Nursing homes first appeared in the nineteenth century and increased in number during the twentieth. Though some functioned well, problems were common enough that anyone who looked could spot them. But it wasn't in anyone's interest to look, not before tens of thousands of patients transferred out of mental hospitals and into nursing homes. Neither psychiatry's leaders nor the government had an interest in looking where these people were headed, as long as it was out the hospital door. Psychiatry could revamp their facilities and recover from the sting of scandal. States liked the idea of shifting costs from state hospitals to less regulated and less expensive nursing homes, especially when that switch came along with federal funding. Nursing home operators welcomed the increase in business. And that increase was massive. In the 1960s, the nursing home population doubled.[18] By the 1980s, there were ten times as many people living in nursing homes as in mental hospitals.[19] Elders with dementia went out one institutional door and in another.

In an ideal world, a big policy shift might include asking the people affected about what they needed and liked. This policy shift did not occur in that ideal world, but in the hurried and harsh real one. Nobody said to patients with dementia, "Please tell me how you're doing. Tell me what would help. Or if you can't tell me, let's have a good look at you and try to put together a batch of helpful things that we can then test to see if they improve your lot." The views of the elderly with dementia, shifted from one involuntary institutional home to another, are lost. Perhaps they wanted to leave the hospital, though for many it had been home for decades. Perhaps their dementia was so advanced they were unaware of their new surroundings. Either way, no one asked them.

Bruce Vladeck, in his excellent 1980 study of the nursing home's history and flaws, argues that federal legislators had very little interest in or understanding of nursing homes before they unleashed the flood of Medicaid and Medicare funds beginning in 1965.[20] But their growth had ramped up even before these entitlement programs, thanks to a series of federal laws. The Hill-Burton Act, amended in 1954, greatly increased funds to build them.[21] Within a few years, there were 10,000 new ones, housing more than 400,000 residents, with an accompanying mammoth surge in costs. Vendor payments to nursing homes had increased tenfold in the five years *before* Medicare and Medicaid got rolling. In 1963, a congressional subcommittee was already preparing a report on the unacceptable conditions of many nursing homes.[22] They varied in size, in patient population, and in level and quality of care. Many were small mom-and-pop operations, with a few rooms in what was once a private home. Licensing requirements were minimal. Many lacked fire prevention measures and accessible exits, a disaster in waiting for elders with limited mobility. Lax food safety and the perennial desire to cut corners meant food could be unpalatable, scant, and occasionally poisonous. Nevertheless, nursing homes were tapped to take over the burden that mental hospitals once carried, the responsibility of caring for isolated, impoverished elders, including those with dementia.

Congress did worry about the potential costs of care for vast numbers of older Americans, so they set up some limits. Medicaid would cover long-term nursing costs, but only for those with low incomes. Medicare would cover elders regardless of their income, but only for shorter stays, mostly for those who were ready to leave the hospital but not sufficiently recovered to go home. The Social Security Administration estimated costs for the first year of Medicare's coverage of these limited nursing home stays at $25 million to $50 million. What could go wrong?

Everything went wrong, just every damn thing. The actual costs for that first year came in at $275 million, ten times the estimate.[23] Every assumption was wrong. First, Social Security administrators knew that few nursing homes met the updated stricter standards, so they figured only a small number of beds were available. Wrong! Other federal apparatchiks, worried about the lack of beds in the face of a new entitlement, created a marvelous loophole. If a nursing home failed to meet standards but was anywhere near close and expressed an endearing intention to improve, then it would fall into the elastic category of "substantial compliance." This creative interpretation of regulatory standards abolished the bed shortage as with a magic wand. Costs would not be limited by the number of beds actually meeting those standards. Not at all. The goalposts were set so far apart it was hard *not* to score Medicare funding.

Second, administrators assumed the Medicare nursing home benefit would save health care dollars by permitting a speedier discharge from an expensive hospital bed to the less costly nursing home bed. Wrong. There was no evidence, none at all, to support this theory. Essentially the opposite occurred. In the blink of an eye, the option of a brief rehabilitative nursing home stay, courtesy of Medicare, morphed into standard care. Now every elderly hospital patient stopped off in a nursing facility on the way home. If the spot wasn't immediately available, the patient would cool her heels in the expensive acute care hospital while waiting. Costs skyrocketed.[24]

Finally, regulators failed to foresee the shocking degree of corruption brought on by these entitlements. Limousines, yachts, slush funds, bribes—all these and more emerged from the nursing home scandals of the 1970s. Frail demented elders were no longer unwanted, but they still weren't seen as deserving of empathic care and a safe harbor. No indeed.

I magine a thief in the 1970s who seeks a business opportunity. Circling like a bird of prey, he spots thousands of people who can't think clearly or remember well and can't contact authorities, and best of all, their pockets connect directly to the deep pockets of the federal government. Our thief spies the frail elders of America, and to him they look like fat and juicy field mice. He swoops in, opening a for-profit nursing home.[25]

Between 1969 and 1975, New York nursing home operators bilked Medicaid of an estimated $42 million.[26] Stealing that much money required ingenuity. The federal government had agreed to reimburse "reasonable costs" but neglected to define "reasonable." Some over-billed for services never rendered or with absurdly inflated costs, but they were much more creative than just that. Fraud rose nearly to an art form. One proprietor bought himself a Renoir for $60,000, then got the vendor to bill him for four hundred imaginary, less expensive artworks to brighten up his nursing homes.[27] Kickbacks were very popular: Among the top thirty local suppliers of nursing home goods and services, they amounted to from 5 to 33 percent of monthly billings.[28]

Medicaid permitted residents to keep a small "personal needs allowance" of $25 per month. These were a delightful source of pocket money, though for administrators rather than residents. One scheme, reminiscent of a bad sitcom, involved a nursing home in which the owners reported *many* armed robberies, always occurring at night when a single employee was on duty, in which the perpetrators could never access the safe with the nursing home's petty cash, but repeatedly popped open and emptied the safe holding the residents' accounts.[29] How terrible!

Real estate manipulation offered enticing options for fleecing the government as well. A home could grossly overestimate its property value, and with it the associated mortgage and depreciation. Nursing home owners made more money if they leased their facility than if they owned it themselves. Dummy corporations concealing ownership sprouted like mushrooms in a bosky glade. Vladeck compares the prevailing ethos to that of a medieval army that was paid subsistence wages—plus all they could steal.[30]

State officials struggled to shut down these shenanigans, but it wasn't easy. In one report, you almost hear the prosecutor pull out his hair over a perp who had evaded justice. This nursing home proprietor received a subpoena demanding access to his books and records in April 1975. Though not a staunch defender of the law *before* receiving the subpoena, he learned to wield it like Poseidon's mighty trident. He brought a motion to quash the subpoena, which he lost. He then lost in the Appellate Division, the New York State Court of Appeals, the Federal District Court, the Federal Circuit Court of Appeals, and the US Supreme Court. At that point he had managed to stay out of prison for two and a half years. An exasperated (and loquacious) judge told him: "Books and records, unlike some ill-starred vessels sailing in the Bermuda triangle, do not disappear without explanation upon the presentation of a subpoena from a Special Prosecutor." Our resilient perp pressed on with the appeals process, losing at every stage but preserving his freedom until April 1978. He spent a few months in jail and then petitioned for release. He still did not have the books. With irrefutable logic, he refused to state why he didn't have them because that might incriminate him. He was released. The prosecutor nearly wept: as of that 1978 report, the owner had yet to find the books, go back to jail, or pay any penalty.[31]

You might think this level of douchebaggery was as low as a perpetrator of Medicaid fraud could go, but you would be wrong. That bottom-of-the-barrel award goes to a Mr. Hochberg, convicted in 1978 of receiving unlawful fees and payments and trying to influence an election, all while he was not only a member of the New York State

Assembly but chair of its Ethics Committee.[32] You can't make this stuff up.

All of these costs, real and fraudulent, tallied up to quite a bill for Medicaid and Medicare. Government officials writhed in shame; their vengeance was swift and fierce. They took many steps to reduce government payments, but the most infamous was the retroactive denial of claims for Medicare beneficiaries. In 1968, the rate of claim denial for extended care was 1.5 percent. As the scope of cost overruns emerged, that rate shot up, so that by 1970 it reached 8.2 percent. Families were left with bills for thousands of dollars for care they thought was guaranteed by the government. Some elders were billed massive amounts, and discharged from nursing homes with no place else to go.[33]

A mess this big helps make change. This one changed the way our government looked at older people. We have the scammers to thank, in a way. Many factors brought dementia to public attention, but a significant contribution came from the nursing home scandals. Those in charge of health policy finally could see the vulnerable elders in their communities, many of them with dementia. What they saw was how shockingly expensive these people were. Theft and abuse could be reduced but not eliminated. Even with better oversight, elders might remain the very expensive guests of government. What on earth could be done with them?

We arrive here at a variant of the care/cure problem. Physicians saw no potential for cure, thus no need for treatment. Such people "only" needed care. When people with dementia left mental hospitals for nursing homes, the goal was to provide "custodial" care at the lowest possible cost. *Custodial* can refer to what a janitor does, and that connotation is relevant here. When a person appears to be beyond cure, medicine has a habit of losing interest. Incurable illness provides few research questions and nothing to add luster to an ambitious career. Cure gets the glory and the big bucks. Care is dull and unremitting, not scientific, not worth paying for. We still bear the consequences of this dichotomy. We've made some gains, but we're not there yet.

Once Medicare and Medicaid are well established, by the 1970s, the demented elders of America are no longer invisible. Now they are seen by predators and payers as either a paycheck or a bill. And then, just as they come into focus, new developments in science—and in the politics of science—hint at a possible solution.

The nursing home debacle was not the only reason this era saw a shift in how the country viewed older people. More people were living into old age, which promoted the growing field of geriatrics and helped change attitudes in important ways.[34] Medical research had gotten a huge boost after World War II. Senator Lyndon Johnson and President Truman suffered heart attacks while in office, and this got the attention of legislators. The idea of promoting medical research with federal dollars gained traction, and indeed became one of the Big Ideas that defined the United States in the second half of the twentieth century.

But the study of dementia faced hurdles that cancer and heart disease did not. Many people, including many physicians, failed to view it as a fatal illness (a failure that persists today, but had not even been flagged as an error at the time). Physicians saw dementia as an end-state for some people, an ill-defined, unfortunate aspect of getting old; it was not yet a separate and distinct illness. Patients with dementia died, but that was because they were debilitated in other ways. One expected them to be carried away by pneumonia, a broken hip, or some other complication of old age; it scarcely mattered which. There was still little research into the topic; rare articles appeared in psychiatric journals, but these were few and far between.[35]

In the 1970s, scientists rediscovered dementia. The electron microscope created images at the level of the cell—an advance of extraordinary impact. Biological research into brain disease gathered steam. My home institution, Albert Einstein College of Medicine in the Bronx, was one of the hubs of the renewed study of dementia. Saul Korey, chair of Neurology, recruited a dynamic group of scientists, including young pathologist Bob Terry, betting that his increasingly refined images from the electron microscope could improve investigations of neuropathology.[36] The two hit it off and began to seek unanswered questions to tackle with their combined expertise. They explored a neurology text and found, near the start of the alphabet, Alzheimer's disease. As far as they knew, no other researchers were planning to take on this illness, and that added to the thrill of the work.[37] Despite research by Solomon Fuller and others in the early 1900s noting that plaques and tangles were not limited to mid-life adults with early onset dementia, this knowledge had been essentially lost. In the 1960s, Alzheimer's was still described in standard texts as a rare illness affecting adults in their forties to sixties, quite distinct from the common dementia that attacked elders. It had become a scientific backwater, but all that was about to change. Terry already had a small grant for "a minor fishing expedition" on the disease; he later learned this was the first NIH grant ever awarded to study Alzheimer's.

The electron microscope revealed minute cellular structures that had never been visible before. Vexing, intriguing questions of structure and function began to unfold. Terry was the first to identify the composition of amyloid plaques. A lively debate about the architecture of tangled neurofibrils emerged; the clear winner was Michael Kidd, who documented that they were double helices.[38] The team at Einstein continued to grow, with Robert Katzman joining the faculty of neurology in 1957. In time, Katzman would chair Neurology while Terry chaired Pathology. Their intellectual dynamism and rigor helped them recruit additional talented researchers, including Peter Davies and Leon Thal.[39]

This nidus of researchers made Einstein in the 1970s an exhilarating place to be. Peter Davies, now a celebrated neuroscientist in his own right, came to Einstein from Scotland when he was still in his twenties. Davies described Bob Terry to me as "a dynamic, aggressive character. He was feared. He was intensely critical. Really *very* sharply critical of anything he thought was the slightest bit substandard."[40]

I commented, "Sounds like it could be scary to be a young researcher in that context."

Davies paused and then said, "Ah . . . it was *wonderful!* I learned it was just always constructive criticism. He didn't want to break you down. He wanted you to defend what you thought. You *should* be able to defend what your viewpoint was. You were a scientist! You better have the data to back your viewpoint. Otherwise, *what* are you doing? What are you saying?"

When Davies saw Terry at a meeting, decades later, they agreed that this period at Einstein was the most stimulating time of their lives. It was a time when sparks flew, when it seemed the answers to great questions were very nearly in their grasp. You can hear in Davies's description the love of the intellectual hunt that defines a great scientist, and the love of science itself.

The restless energy, the discoveries, the formal and informal exchanges about cutting-edge science kept this coterie of researchers on their toes. But science was not the only domain in which they excelled. Katzman in particular discovered a talent for public advocacy and the political aspects of science. He is widely recognized for his 1976 editorial in the *Archives of Neurology*, in which he laid out the terrifying demographics of dementia, with the projected increase in the population of older people and the disease in the approaching decades.[41] While the standard usage at the time defined Alzheimer's as a rare form of dementia for midlife adults, he stated that neither clinicians nor pathologists had any way of distinguishing between Alzheimer's in these younger patients and Alzheimer-type dementia in patients in their sixties and beyond. (Fuller had, of course, observed this overlap decades before.) The brain pathology and the symptoms were the same. Worse, far from being rare, including both young and older persons made dementia, by Katzman's estimate, the fourth or fifth largest killer in the United States.[42] Katzman was a more than capable scientist, but this editorial was not about science. It was about changing the definition of dementia. It demanded that when physicians looked at dementia, they recognize an entity they had not properly seen before. He wanted physicians to see it as an illness in the elderly that was widespread, deadly, and a crucial public health challenge. He changed the game.

Katzman was not content merely to publish this rabble-rousing editorial in a medical journal. He wanted to tip the scale of funding for research. He would goad the federal government into action. To do that, he would work the levers of democracy by creating a public outcry. And to do that, he would partner with families and patients. Katzman himself was eloquent in describing the suffering of those with dementia and the need for more funding. He also knew that a grieving spouse could deliver that message like a hand grenade. He helped create the Alzheimer's Association, work that made him as proud as anything else he accomplished in his long career.

But that career was not always at Einstein, where longstanding tensions erupted. A psychiatrist who was the new hospital president, Carl

Eisdorfer, hoped to make a glorious triumvirate with Katzman and Terry, who respectively chaired Neurology and Pathology. Katzman and Terry rejected his efforts at collaboration. Katzman and Terry knew they were brilliant, and pretty much everyone else agreed. They didn't see Eisdorfer's research as on par with what they could do.[43] Was it psychiatry they didn't like, or a type of psychiatric research or a particular psychiatrist? It's hard to know. In any event, Terry and Katzman did not see why they should work with someone they didn't choose to work with. Eisdorfer responded, reportedly, by making their lives a living hell. Mediation was attempted in an effort to preserve reasonable working relationships among the various people and departments.[44] No go; in 1984 Katzman and Terry moved, lock, stock, and two smoking barrels, to the University of California at San Diego. Even today, their colleagues at Einstein are sad about their departure. Not long after Katzman and Terry left, Eisdorfer was shown the door.[45] Change was in the air, not just at Einstein but for every aspect of this new field of research.

Forces had gathered from vastly different sectors to pull dementia into the light. The cost of care ballooned, and those costs moved front and center in the national policy agenda. Scientific advances made it possible to study the disease in ways unthinkable a decade earlier. And then a group of dynamic, effective advocates came together in Washington, DC, to give the final necessary push for dementia's arrival.

Chapter 6

Princesses and Presidents: Dementia Rebranded

Florence Mahoney was a pistol, as my grandmother would have said. Born in 1899 near Muncie, Indiana, Florence rejected the standard pathways for young women of that time and came to wield great influence in national politics. In her teens, she set out alone for Moose Jaw, Saskatchewan, defying her father's wishes, and landed her first job teaching dance and physical activities at the YWCA. She was a hit there, leading local girls in public demonstrations of youth and agility while still a girl herself. Though rebellious, she was consistent. Mahoney was a lifelong enthusiast for the health benefits of exercise until she died at 103.

Mahoney and her close friend Mary Lasker strong-armed politicians and other decision-makers in Washington over decades, leaving an indelible imprint on the National Institutes of Health and on research in cancer and diseases of the aging. Jack Valenti, then assistant to President Lyndon Johnson, claimed, "When I would tell him that

Mary Lasker and Florence Mahoney wanted to see him, the president would groan. He'd say, 'Oh, my God, these two women are going to bankrupt the country.' And they usually got what they wanted out of him."[1]

Both Lasker and Mahoney were lively and gracious, yet the two friends had different methods of persuasion. Lasker had vast wealth, estimated at more than $80 million in the 1960s. That wealth was a potent weapon, used strategically. Most notably, she and her husband, Albert Lasker, created the Lasker Awards, which reward scientists for significant discoveries and contributions to public health.[2] The prize included very welcome funding, but also unbeatable publicity. Lasker Award winners often go on to win Nobel Prizes, and so the Lasker offers its winner the mantle of yet greater things to come. Not all Lasker Awards went to scientists. Some went to elected officials for their service to health-related causes. Brilliantly, Lasker once awarded the award to two champions of hers, in the Senate and the House, who had fallen into feuding. These leaders, Senator Lister Hill and Congressman John Fogarty, settled back into a pattern of helpful support for her projects after receiving their awards.

Florence Mahoney's influence was less direct. She had little formal education in science. She was affluent, but not on the scale of Mary Lasker. Mahoney married and later divorced Dan Mahoney, the publisher of the Cox newspapers, a successful chain with wide distribution. She raised her sons in an elegant beachfront home in Miami, and summered with them on her ranch in Idaho. She collected Chinese porcelains admired by Jackie Kennedy. But she would not have been able to fund a prestigious prize and did not make significant campaign contributions. What resources she had, she used to excellent effect. She was an early savant on the value of publicity. Long after her divorce, she was still able to offer elected officials newspaper coverage and strongly favorable editorials that reached constituents. A positive editorial in the *Miami Daily News* meant a lot, including to Senator Claude Pepper, who was often encouraged with just such coverage.[3]

But publicity was not Mahoney's primary weapon. Her true artistry was in networking, which had not even been named at that point. She was utterly comfortable engaging anyone in conversation, no matter how famous. Spying Winston Churchill walking on the beach near her Florida home, she marched right up to him and asked about a physician whose unorthodox ideas interested her. Churchill labeled the man a crackpot and gave Mahoney a jovial slap on the back that nearly knocked her to the ground.[4] She took the backslap in stride. It would take more than that to shut her down.

Mahoney's true skills emerged after her divorce in 1950, when she moved to Washington and set herself up in a modest but pretty Georgetown town house. She took to hosting dinner parties of six to eight people; these became the most desirable invitations in a town where invitations mattered. The small parties may have in part reflected economic constraints, but they produced a big impact. She aimed to bring together specific people. While these connections furthered her own aims, they were at least as useful to the guests. She had a knack for befriending Democratic presidents and their wives. She was on close, informal terms with the families of Truman, Kennedy, and Johnson, regularly dining in the White House during these administrations, both at big state dinners as well as in intimate family settings.

That access was a golden prize for the young strivers she collected. Consider the good fortune of Joe English, a doctor who ran various antipoverty programs in the Johnson administration.[5] When English showed up to dinner at Mahoney's one evening with a long face, she pulled out of him the information that funds for a treasured program of his were blocked. She went right to the phone, and English could hear her say that "this young doctor has all these good programs—it's just what your husband is wanting to do; it may be the most important health program in the administration, but it could go down the tubes." Lady Bird Johnson, on the other end, reassured Mahoney, who in turn told English not to worry. The next morning the president's press secretary phoned him, rather surprised, to say that English's program had just been selected as one of the Johnson administration's five showcase pieces of legislation. Mahoney didn't have to tell English that he owed her. Rather, she made of him a lifelong fan. Throughout her career she went out of her way to promote talented young people, even while she befriended those higher up the food chain. She never took credit. She got things done.

Mahoney influenced health policy on many issues throughout her long career as an unpaid lobbyist. For years, she and Mary Lasker worked together and took vacations together, arriving in Hawaii or other scenic spots to enjoy the surroundings and continue their plotting. But her greatest project, and greatest victory, she carried out without Lasker's assistance. Mahoney is generally acknowledged as the driving force behind the creation of the National Institute on Aging (NIA). She did not work alone, of course, but without her persistence, the NIA would not have come into being as and when it did.

Mahoney served on an advisory council for the National Institute of Child Health and Human Development. Officially, this institute was to look at diseases across the life-span, but in practice it focused on children. Mahoney was annoyed that grants related to aging were consistently rejected. Over time, she became convinced of the need for an institute focused on diseases of aging. Few agreed. The Association of American Medical Colleges, which had supported the creation of a number of institutes, came out against it. But Mahoney kept at it, year after year. She could, as they say, talk a dog off a meat truck.

Mahoney was in her seventies by then and still a blur of activity. She sized up a newly minted Senator Thomas Eagleton, chair of a new subcommittee on aging. She encouraged him at one of her dinners to sponsor the legislation. He too became a lifelong collaborator of hers. The legislation passed both the House and Senate in 1972, and was sent to President Nixon for his signature.

But the NIA had a difficult birth. Nixon, troubled by budget deficits, disliked adding another institute to the growing number at NIH. He vetoed that legislation. Other opponents included Dr. Merlin K. DuVal, assistant secretary of Health, Education and Welfare, who argued "there is little basis for separating this activity from research on the same disease when it afflicts the young or middle aged. To do so would cause the almost inevitable result of duplicative work at two or more institutes, merely because a disease, such as cancer, can affect persons at many age levels."[6] During House floor debate, H. R. Gross, Republican of Iowa, voted against the bill, bloviating that "We do not need to spend millions of dollars, so far as I am concerned, to tell me that I am getting older as the days go by."[7]

These powerful men didn't know the force they were up against. The legislation authorizing NIA was passed by both the House and Senate again in 1973 and sent to Nixon, who declined to sign it. Still, legislators, a growing coalition of scientists, citizen groups, and always Mahoney kept at it. The bill was passed again in 1974. By that point, Nixon had bigger fish to fry. Months from leaving office, he chose not to waste energy on another veto and signed the NIA into life in May 1974. Mahoney conquered.

The new institute needed someone to run it. NIH funds scientific research, so a scientific researcher would be first choice. But what looked like a plum job had drawbacks for those qualified to hold it. Taking on a weighty administrative burden is a proven method for keeping scientists out of their labs, and they don't like that. The candidacy of a prominent Stanford researcher was derailed by an ugly lawsuit about who could bag the profit from a discovery developed with NIH funding.[8] The search for a director lurched along, and then Robert Butler, author of a popular book advocating for elders, swung into view.

Butler was not a typical candidate to lead an institute at NIH, for he was more of a clinician than a researcher. He had started his career as a psychiatrist in the early years of the National Institute of Mental Health (NIMH), where he did part of his training. After leaving NIMH, Butler continued to see patients, sharpening his clinical skills. He did not do laboratory research; his most famous innovation is the life review, in which an older person recalls events across the life-span to reestablish a sense of meaning and continuity. Though still widely used in clinical social work, this was not the hard science research that NIH generally looked for. Still, Butler had other skills and a special affinity for older people. He advocated for better care in nursing homes and started a day program in a nursing home basement, helping "people who were bedfast or chairfast come alive with the opportunity to mix with other people."[9] Living in Washington, DC, he paired his medical expertise with political engagement. He served as a delegate to the infamous 1968 Democratic National Convention in Chicago, observing firsthand the clashes of demonstrators and police. He used his growing and highly effective social network to change policy on a broader level. He became a public intellectual.

Butler's ideas often found their way into print, not only in scholarly journals but also in the widely read popular media. In 1969, he coined the term *ageism*, defined as a "systemic stereotyping of and discrimination against old people because they are old, just as racism and sexism accomplish this with skin color and gender."[10] The word filled an important need, making explicit the link between the movement to protect the rights of elders, and the movements to protect the rights of minorities. Butler's word was quoted in *The Washington Post* by Carl Bernstein and was incorporated into the *Oxford English Dictionary*.[11] His creativity won him notoriety; it did not hurt that among his friends were many prominent journalists. Robert C. Maynard, the first African American member of the editorial board of the *Post*, was one of his closest friends. They were neighbors, they ran together, they taught courses together. Maynard married his wife at Butler's house.[12] Through Maynard, Butler met other prominent journalists. His network included scientists and government officials as well. Butler was a gregarious, energetic, generous man. His broad network of friends and colleagues helped build his public platform.

For all these reasons, Butler was already well-known in Washington's interlocking power circles of science, government, and media when he published *Why Survive?: Being Old in America*,[13] the Pulitzer Prize winner for nonfiction in 1976. The book and Butler himself were discussed everywhere, in print and in private gatherings. He raged against the practices and policies that made old age so much more terrible than necessary. Among his many impressed readers was Florence Mahoney.

Having Mahoney in his corner was a very good thing for Butler. When she had the thought that Butler would make a suitable leader, she knew how to get that thought a hearing in the right places. She talked up his name through her chain of contacts, landing it directly in the path of the new director of NIH, Dr. Donald S. Fredrickson, as well as the chair of the search committee, Dr. Ronald W.

Lamont-Havers.[14] They knew of Mahoney's role in getting NIA funded. Butler was named the first director of the NIA.

But NIA's troubles, and Butler's, were far from over. NIA had won the struggle to exist, but that didn't mean opposition had vanished, or that sibling institutes at NIH would happily share resources with the new baby. To the contrary, NIA's first budget amounted to only 1 percent of NIH funding, or less than $20 million.[15] As opponents had noted, other institutes were already looking at many diseases that affected the elderly, including heart disease, mental illness, and cancer. Butler needed to assure NIA's survival, and he would need more funds to do that. But he would never succeed in getting money to duplicate or compete with ongoing work at NIH. The institute was trapped in a circular prison: To get more funding, they had to add value. To add value, they needed more money. They needed a special research focus relevant to older people, one important enough to wring new funding out of the federal government and that no one else was working on.

Butler's task was tough, but he had one especially effective weapon: Zaven Khachaturian, who would later become known as the father of Alzheimer's research. Back then, Khachaturian was young and had covered a lot of territory on the way to NIH.[16] He has a deep, gravelly voice and a fairly thick accent, one that is hard to place, but that does not disguise the brilliance of what he has to say. As it turns out, he is from a lot of places. Khachaturian was born in Aleppo, Syria, to an Armenian family. Like countless others, they were driven from their home during the Armenian genocide, in which the Ottoman government rounded up and killed an estimated 1.5 million men, women, and children toward the end of World War I. His family lived in Syria between the world wars, while the French ruled, and left when the French left. This time they went to Beirut, Lebanon, where young Zaven lived through high school. He then left for the United States, where he gained admission to Yale College, no easy feat for a refugee from Syria, by way of Beirut, with an accent and a funny name. Yale had made a sound choice. Khatchaturian's appetite for learning was voracious. He started with the Greek philosophers and then investigated biology, chemistry, learning, and memory. He earned a PhD in neurophysiology at Case Western Reserve University, pursued a postdoc at Columbia, and then joined the research faculty at the University of Pittsburgh. By then it was the 1970s, and Khachaturian added an interest in public policy. He had learned the hard way that funding was tight. He set out to learn who made decisions about research and the money that made it possible.

As a faculty member at Pittsburgh, he could take courses, and so he did, studying legislative history, the federal budget process, and "a lot of nitty-gritty of public policy."[17] He then heard of an even better learning opportunity: NIH had just started a one-year training program in public policy. Off he went to Washington. The program assigned the participants a mentor and sent trainees to offices in various parts of the federal government—three weeks here and a month there—where they learned firsthand who made decisions and how. He worked for the secretary of HEW, Joseph Califano. He worked for the congressional subcommittee that passed most of the laws relevant to public health. He learned how a proposal got to a decision-maker, who made decisions at each level of government, and what led to a favorable decision. He was the Willie Sutton of health policy. He studied the government because that's where the money was. He mastered the process that puts federal funds into a researcher's hand. He amassed all the data needed to build a strategy for shepherding a research program through the wilderness of the federal funding apparatus.

One of Khachaturian's assignments was to the nascent NIA and the office of Robert Butler. Their skills and approach were well-balanced, and their goals overlapped. Butler was a superb clinician, with a passion for improving the lot of older people. He wanted to change the public's ideas about aging, and he wanted to help NIA survive by building a robust research program. Khachaturian wanted to use his newfound knowledge to win funds and see what he could build. He needed someone to tell a compelling clinical story to get the wheels of government and science turning. Their plans intersected at Alzheimer's disease. Butler asked Khachaturian to develop a strategic plan to build a research program in brain aging and Alzheimer's. Butler liked what he saw. He hired Khachaturian to stay at NIA and implement his strategy.

All the pieces were coming together. A crew of brilliant researchers looked at the neuropathology of Alzheimer's and found an intriguing unsolved puzzle. The director of a new national institute was looking for an important disease related to aging that was insufficiently studied, around which to build a research program. A scientist with a keen sense of strategy was right there, at the NIH, looking to build just such a program. There was just one more piece missing, but it was a crucial one, needed to drive the engine of funding for the research program. They needed a public voice, demanding that the government do something about Alzheimer's. This piece, which took the form of the Alzheimer's Association, was the most powerful ingredient in the mix. It created enough energy to light up dementia and show it to the world.

Like an elephant, the Alzheimer's Association had a long gestation. Its creators include many of the same characters who helped form the NIA. Robert Katzman had mused about the benefit of a consumer group as early as 1974.[18] Robert Butler, impressed by Katzman's celebrated 1976 editorial, helped organize a symposium on Alzheimer's disease at NIH. There, Butler, Katzman, and others discussed the need for a public advocacy group; Katzman kept the idea moving forward.

By December 1978, New York attorney Lonnie Wollin, volunteering his services, had incorporated the Alzheimer Disease Society and arranged its nonprofit status.

Florence Mahoney, force of nature, had helped launch NIA by talking until she beat the opposition down. Once the institute was up and running, Mahoney kept talking, including to Robert Butler, who owed her his directorship. She encouraged Butler to reach out to Jerome Stone, a wealthy Chicago businessman who ran his family's packaging business.[19] Stone's wife, Evelyn, had been diagnosed with Alzheimer's in 1970. Stone was amazed at how difficult it had been to find out what was wrong. Their family doctor thought Evelyn suffered from "a little bit of depression." The family was advised to "just give her a lot of loving and affection and everything will be all right. Common . . . in women whose children have left the nest."[20] Stone was dismayed by how little the disease was understood and how little was available to help his wife. Mahoney recognized the perfect leader for an advocacy group: Stone was motivated, effective, wealthy, and well connected. She applied her special brand of fingerspitzengefühl, a deft, light touch that helped people see that the direction she wanted them to take was where they'd wanted to go all along. She helped Jerome Stone see that he wanted to be one of the country's first family advocates for Alzheimer's disease.

By March 1979, Robert Terry had invited Stone to join the board of the newly formed "society dedicated to Alzheimer's Disease."[21] Terry notes wistfully that the society has neither funds nor an office, and hopes that he will help get things rolling. In May, Katzman wrote Stone, who had already agreed to join the board.[22] Katzman lays out the goals he has in mind for the new organization, listing education and assistance for patients and family members. Yet he makes crystal clear that the "major objective of the Society . . . is to support research in

Alzheimer's disease and related disorders both by giving direct research support to scientists and by using whatever leverage may be developed to help increase the National Institutes of Health budgets for this disease."[23] (These various goals, and their differential importance to the group, will lead to tensions that never quite go away, even up to the present day.) By September 1979, representatives of several groups interested in dementia gathered in Minnesota to discuss the advantages of forming a national association.[24] They met next at NIH, under the sponsorship of Butler, joined by Stone and others, with the express purpose of creating a national organization, which named itself the Alzheimer's Disease and Related Diseases Association (ADRDA).

All this time, Florence Mahoney kept talking. She gave Stone the contact information for Nick Cavarocchi, a fledgling lobbyist she'd met when he worked on the House Appropriations Committee. With her keen grasp of human motivation, she also pointed out to Cavarocchi that by helping Stone, he would get his business well launched.[25] The first official meeting of ADRDA took place in December 1979, at the Chicago offices of Stone's company. In attendance were locally and nationally prominent businesspeople and philanthropists, board members, and Dominic Ruscio, Cavarocchi's partner, a former Capitol Hill staffer for the Senate Appropriations Committee. Ruscio was used to working with "kitchen-table patient advocacy groups" yearning for a meeting with their congressman. Stone operated at a different level altogether. Before starting in on the official agenda, he observed that ADRDA needed funding for staff and offices. They needed lots of money—$50,000. Instantly, the new board members took out their checkbooks and met the need. This took Ruscio's breath away—in his budding lobbyist career, he had never seen anything like this. Stone then calmly moved on to the formal agenda.[26]

The organization wasted no time. Following Mahoney's policy, they started at the top. By July 1980, they were working with Senator Eagleton, a sponsor of the legislation that created NIA. Eagleton now organized a congressional hearing on Alzheimer's disease, featuring testimony from Stone, Butler, and others. It is hard to believe today, but at that time almost no one outside of an elite circle of scientists and advocates had ever heard of Alzheimer's. A guide for wary travelers was needed. Looking over a senator's shoulder at one hearing, an observer read an index card with this pronunciation guide: *Altz'-hi-merz* and *de-'men-sha*.[27] These congressional hearings explored unknown territory.

At the national level, ADRDA tackled the difficult work of educating decision-makers, stressing that Alzheimer's was a specific disease and not an inevitable consequence of aging. Local offshoots were starting up, affiliated with the umbrella organization. By the end of 1980 there were twenty chapters and a national office in New York. The organization was a loose federation, with local chapters organizing activities, many focused on support for family caregivers. ("What is a rap session?" read one early newsletter, encouraging family members to come in and discuss the challenges of caring for a loved one with Alzheimer's.)[28] In those days before the internet, information was in short supply, so ADRDA developed an information booklet for patients and family members.

Even with all this momentum, ADRDA was gobsmacked by its first real dose of publicity. On October 23, 1980, *Dear Abby* published a letter from "Desperate in NY."[29] Identical twin advice columnists Abby and Ann Landers (really Pauline Esther "Popo" Phillips and Esther Pauline "Eppie" Lederer, respectively) had been described as "the most widely read and most quoted women in the world."[30] "Desperate" wrote about baffling changes in her husband over the past two years. He was only fifty years old and suffered grievous deterioration in memory and function. He lost his job; he could no longer drive. She couldn't leave him alone in the house. After visiting many doctors, he received a diagnosis of Alzheimer's. Desperate wrote, "Have you ever heard of Alzheimer's Disease? I feel so helpless. How do others cope with this affliction?" Abby hit this one out of the park. Having written to NIH for information, she responded to Desperate with a brief paragraph describing newly organized groups of friends and relatives who offered support and information. She told Desperate to send a stamped, self-addressed envelope to ADRDA, at an address on lower Broadway in New York City.

This brief comment in *Dear Abby* caught ADRDA off guard—and the public's embrace nearly crushed the infant organization. Desperate must have been one of the 35,000 people who asked for information in the weeks following publication of the letter. Demand quickly outstripped available booklets; the NIA stepped in and printed additional copies. Alzheimer's was no longer obscure. People across the country had seen these signs in themselves and their loved ones, and were hungry for more information. *Dear Abby* had launched Alzheimer's disease into the public consciousness. Sadly, this was not her last encounter with the disease. She drafted her daughter as an assistant in writing the column until, in 2002, Jeanne took over the Dear Abby pen name, column, and associated media enterprises completely. The reason: Pauline had been diagnosed with Alzheimer's.[31]

ADRDA survived the onslaught of attention, growing rapidly stronger and more visible. The highly effective combination of unpaid lobbyist Mahoney and paid lobbyists Cavarocchi and Ruscio capitalized on each success, talking more dogs off more meat trucks. They built an impressive record of supporters on Capitol Hill and elsewhere who knew about Alzheimer's and wanted to help conquer it. Their methods were creative and effective. Cavarocchi and Ruscio noted that in those days women were in relatively short supply on Capitol

Hill, while the vast majority of elected representatives were older men, many of them World War II veterans. What better way to get their attention than to send a beautiful woman into their midst? And what better woman could there be than one closely related to Rita Hayworth, every World War II vet's favorite pinup? So it was that the Alzheimer's Association, working with its board and lobbyists, persuaded Princess Yasmin Aga Khan, daughter of Rita Hayworth, to testify before Congress regarding Alzheimer's, starting in 1982.

Hayworth, unluckily for her, was one of the first celebrities diagnosed with Alzheimer's. As was true of many with dementia at the time (and still too many today), her symptoms went unrecognized for years. Her cognitive decline, erratic behavior, and memory loss were attributed to alcoholism, and her image was tarnished. Her daughter wished to both restore her mother's reputation and help her and other patients. Like her mother, Princess Yasmin Aga Khan was a great beauty. As Dom Ruscio put it, "most of the members [of Congress] then were in their sixties, seventies, eighties. You could see them thinking, 'This is the closest I'm ever going to come to Rita Hayworth!'"[32] The princess drew a capacity crowd. She delivered a moving and effective message; the hearing was a huge success. Knowledge of Alzheimer's and research funds kept increasing.

A glowing report to the association's board from Cavarocchi and Ruscio in February 1984 conveys some of the giddy feeling of this victory. The report opens with a quote from Margaret Heckler, Secretary for Health and Human Services, labeling Alzheimer's "a disease of catastrophic proportions." Heckler had delivered her statement during a hearing before the Senate Subcommittee on Aging. She made an even more pleasing statement before she was done, announcing that federal funding for Alzheimer's research would increase that year by nearly another 50 percent.[33]

Heckler's happy announcement was the culmination of a string of prior successes. Among these were the unprecedented twelve congressional hearings on Alzheimer's in that year alone. Even Domenic Ruscio, who had played a major role in orchestrating this success, was surprised by it. But as he went about on Capitol Hill, trying to get in the door to speak with elected officials about Alzheimer's, he kept running into people who had been directly affected by the disease: "I went in to talk with Senator Howard Metzenbaum's staff. I got about three sentences in—I usually had to explain what Alzheimer's was—and the staff member said, 'I know about it already. My husband has it.' And I said, 'Oh! I'm so sorry.' She said, 'Yes, and not only do I understand, but Senator Metzenbaum understands. His roommate from law school has Alzheimer's.'"

Ruscio soon met with Senator Metzenbaum, an influential member of the Budget Committee, whose support was even more emphatic than he had hoped. Metzenbaum was happy to promote funding for research generally, but asked if there was "something more, anything else we could do?" When a senator asks a lobbyist if there is something more he can do, the answer is always yes. Ruscio, thinking quickly and drawing on a fleeting conversation with Katzman, asked for money for centers, multidisciplinary research centers, at different institutions across the country.

The appropriations bill had already come out of committee. Senator Metzenbaum was a canny parliamentarian and had discovered that amendments to existing bills could be used in creative and effective ways. He proposed adding these funds for Alzheimer's research centers as a floor amendment. This additional funding would march along with the larger appropriations bill; if done correctly, it would be easier to pass the larger bill with its amendments than without. Metzenbaum's staff worked to secure support throughout the Senate; the amendment passed. That was the crucial step toward funding the Alzheimer's disease research centers. Ruscio immediately called Katzman, saying, "You're not going to believe this!" Katzman and colleagues went into battle mode, drafting a grant proposal that could be circulated by NIH, requesting applications to create the centers that had just managed, out of the blue, to get funding.

They didn't have to work alone. At NIH they could rely on a helpful "inside man," as Dom Ruscio described Zaven Khachaturian.[34] There were those who wanted to limit NIA's focus on Alzheimer's; there were complaints that NIA was evolving into the "National Institute for Alzheimer's." But Khachaturian was able to negotiate within and outside of NIA and NIH. The grant and the centers succeeded in moving along the tortuous path from Congress through the appropriations process and to the final delivery of research funds to scientists.

Throughout the 1980s, Alzheimer's was in the news and in the public eye. In 1981, Nancy Mace and Peter Rabins published *The 36-Hour Day*, a blockbuster book devoted to supporting family members of those suffering from Alzheimer's—no longer would the public have to rely exclusively on the slim pamphlet provided by the Alzheimer's Association.[35] Now in its sixth edition, the book reigns supreme as the self-help volume for people affected by the disease. By 1982, many major news outlets, including *The New York Times*, *The Washington Post*, *Ladies' Home Journal*, *Good Morning America*, and *Reader's Digest* all provided prominent coverage. President Reagan declared the first National Alzheimer's Disease Awareness Month in 1983. A television movie, *Do You Remember Love*, starred Joanne Woodward as a woman with Alzheimer's and Richard Kiley as her loving husband.

. . .

A nd then the thunderclap. On November 5, 1994, former President Ronald Reagan published an open letter revealing his own recent diagnosis. The letter is both intimate and candid; it is handwritten and clear:

> *My fellow Americans,*
>
> *I have recently been told that I am one of the millions of Americans who will be afflicted with Alzheimer's disease.*
>
> *Upon learning this news, Nancy and I had to decide whether as private citizens we would keep this a private matter or whether we would make this news known in a public way.*
>
> *In the past, Nancy suffered from breast cancer and I had cancer surgeries. We found through our open disclosures we were able to raise public awareness. We were happy that as a result many more people underwent testing. They were treated in early stages and able to return to normal, healthy lives.*
>
> *So now we feel it is important to share it with you. In opening our hearts, we hope this might promote greater awareness of this condition. Perhaps it will encourage a clear understanding of the individuals and families who are affected by it.*
>
> *At the moment, I feel just fine. I intend to live the remainder of the years God gives me on this earth doing the things I have always done. I will continue to share life's journey with my beloved Nancy and my family. I plan to*

*enjoy the great outdoors and stay in touch with my friends
and supporters.*

*Unfortunately, as Alzheimer's disease progresses, the
family often bears a heavy burden. I only wish there was
some way I could spare Nancy from this painful experience.
When the time comes, I am confident that with your help
she will face it with faith and courage.*

*In closing, let me thank you, the American people, for
giving me the great honor of allowing me to serve as your
president. When the Lord calls me home, whenever that may
be, I will leave the greatest love for this country of ours and
eternal optimism for its future.*

*I now begin the journey that will lead me into the sunset
of my life. I know that for America there will always be a
bright dawn ahead.*

Thank you, my friends.[36]

The immediate reaction was an outpouring of sympathy, grief, and
respect. Letters of support flooded into the Reagan home. Even those
who had bitterly opposed Reagan's policies accepted the dignity and
courage of his response to his diagnosis. President Bill Clinton, at a
large rally on the day of the announcement, praised Reagan's "optimism and spirit" and asked the crowd to "give Ronald Reagan a hand
and wish him well."[37] Shortly after the announcement, speculation
began that Reagan had demonstrated cognitive deficits during his
presidency. Certainly reporters and others had noted memory lapses,
and research suggests Reagan's speech patterns at press conferences
became less complex over time.[38] Still, these demonstrated cognitive
deficits don't prove he met the criteria for dementia during his presidential term, which ended eight years before the announcement. The

Reagans continued to promote Alzheimer's awareness. They created the Ronald and Nancy Reagan Research Institute. Nancy Reagan supported Alzheimer's research for the rest of her life, as did their daughter Maureen Reagan.

Alzheimer's had arrived. After Reagan's announcement, it would be tough to find a consumer of news anywhere in the world who had not heard of the disease. In the early 1970s, Alzheimer's had been an obscure malady that required a pronunciation guide. Some doubted that it really was an illness, rather than just an unfortunate and inevitable aspect of aging. Total NIH funding for the disease in 1976 was a mere $3.8 million, small potatoes relative to research funding for other major illnesses. By the turn of the century, NIH funding for Alzheimer's and related dementias was more than $400 million annually, a hundredfold increase. These gains meant that scientists across the country could start to untangle how the brain breaks down in dementia, and what forces are protective or harmful. Alzheimer's disease rode this growing funding stream from utter obscurity to household word. This success was in part due to canny marketing and lobbying by the Alzheimer's Association.[39]

The success of Alzheimer's advocacy relied in large measure on the argument that dementia was a disease, not an inevitable consequence of aging. As Robert Butler wrote, "The public does not see itself as 'suffering' from the basic biology of aging, nor does it generally believe that aging per se can be reversed. Rather the public has come to view medical research as contributing to an understanding of specific diseases associated with old age."[40] There were many who disagreed, finding that dementia was difficult to sort out from the expected process of aging. Indeed, it is not always easy to draw a line between normal cognitive aging and dementia. Similar diagnostic issues arise in a wide range of diseases; kidney function, for example, declines with age, and it is challenging to identify the exact point at which normal decline crosses over into a disease process.

Exchanges on this topic have been quite heated. Katzman took a strong stand, noting, "I have spent a number of years trying to persuade people that Alzheimer's *is* a disease, and not simply what used to be called 'senility' or 'senile dementia.'"[41] Many authors, including Jesse Ballenger and Margaret Lock, have written insightfully about the debate on differentiating normal aging from dementia.[42]

Butler believed he could not succeed in building up NIA with research into the process of aging. There was too much stigma to combat—too many people understood aging, and all its ramifications, as inevitable. Butler needed to advocate for research into specific diseases. These had to have real public health impact and not compete with the efforts of other NIH institutes. Alzheimer's was a perfect fit. Butler promoted research on Alzheimer's as the platform for NIA's success. Helping set up the public advocacy arm to draw attention to Alzheimer's also fit perfectly with this plan.

But this strategy, brilliant though it was, had flaws. Katzman, the most ardent of Alzheimer's boosters, reveals the main problem while describing the inspiration for his famous 1976 editorial: "I looked up some of the epidemiological data that was coming out, that about 50 to 60 percent of the cases had Alzheimer's disease."[43] Katzman is telling us something important here, something that gets swept under the rug in the blitz of marketing to promote Alzheimer's research. Only half of patients with dementia have the plaques and tangles that constitute Alzheimer's pathology. The other half do not.

In the recent past, people with dementia went without any diagnosis. (Recall Jerome Stone's wife, who was told she would be fine with "a lot of love and affection.") Sadly, many patients and families still live in this era; the diagnosis of dementia is routinely missed. Those who do now receive the diagnosis of dementia are generally told they have Alzheimer's disease. Some receive this diagnosis after careful testing and examination, but many are diagnosed after only modest efforts to exclude other causes for cognitive decline. Even today, relatively few receive an evaluation by specialists. Now a person with dementia is likely to be told he or she has Alzheimer's, but until quite recently, there was virtually no way to confirm Alzheimer's in a living person.

Dementia is not a single disease. Like cancer, there are multiple forms, and many people are affected by more than one. The single greatest risk factor for dementia of any sort remains advancing age. But the focus on pathology, necessary though it was, to some degree stalled our efforts to untangle the ways in which aging, multiple other illnesses, and social determinants of health contribute to dementia. Even in those with Alzheimer's, there are often other forms of pathology, including damage from strokes, diabetes, physical trauma, and all the other wear and tear of a long life. This makes the search for a cure far more challenging, for the odds of finding a single pill that will combat the effects of eighty years of life, with the accumulated impact of multiple diseases, are quite remote. Dementia is not an inevitable consequence of aging, but our efforts to make that point led us to neglect the ways in which aging, multiple influences, and dementia are intertwined.[44]

Dementia came of age in the 1970s and 1980s. True, there had been earlier glimpses of dementia, especially in the early twentieth-century efforts to unravel its mysterious brain pathology. Those earlier achievements did not match the sonic boom of attention generated by a princess, a president, and an army of dedicated troops. But just at the moment of its debut, dementia as a family of diseases was overshadowed by a single important, noisy, rich sibling. Alzheimer's disease gets the money and gets the glory. The ADRDA drops the "related diseases" from its title and becomes the Alzheimer's Association. What's in that name change? Only a catchier label or a shift in strategy? The Alzheimer's Association rapidly became a significant player in national health politics, tied in as it was with NIH, key researchers, political clout, and a vast network of membership-driven chapters. But as in many success stories, someone was left behind. The many people with dementia who don't have Alzheimer's did not receive the same outpouring of research dollars and attention.

To pile on a different metaphor, Alzheimer's is the rich donor who buys the right to rename the hospital—it's no longer Memorial Hospital, it's [Your Name Here] Hospital. Just as dementia arrives, it becomes Alzheimer's. This miracle of marketing and political savvy generates much-needed funding, which in turn attracts interest from scientists, more research success, and yet more funders. That's all to the good. But while something is gained, something is lost. While it becomes easier to study Alzheimer's, some say the light that shines there leaves other researchers and other patients, plus important theories and types of pathology, in the dark. Others counter that a rising tide floats all boats. We are still sorting out the consequences of the marketing success of Alzheimer's disease.

Chapter 7

Dementia's Progress

Alzheimer's was on the map. The NIA had triumphed over its opponents and was up and running toward Alzheimer's. Science was gunning its engines, racing to cure dementia. But researchers faced a modern-day secular Pilgrim's Progress. There were still multiple barriers to overcome, three of which we'll examine. Any one of these barriers, if not surmounted, could stop dementia research in its tracks, leaving the field in the Slough of Despond. The first challenge is defining dementia so as to point scientists in the right direction for productive work. The second impediment is the competition for research funding. The third—the most difficult—is "just science," or the unending struggle to solve complex scientific puzzles. None of these barriers is ever entirely overcome, but a full failure in any one halts progress.

Let's start with dementia's definition, a problem that resurfaces in different eras. Once dementia was just old age, a slow turning toward death. Work done during the start of the twentieth century—by Alzheimer, Fuller, and others—showed that dementia was not a generic fading away. Specific cellular changes occurred, though the correlation to symptoms was far from straightforward. Dementia then falls off the to-do list of science for decades. Cardiac disease, cancer—these are where the best minds went, where the scientific prizes waited. Then, as we've seen, dementia steps into the limelight. Now science gets on board, really for the first time, to delve into the problem. But this renewed interest in the 1970s sparks a skirmish in the battle to define what makes a brain disease. The debate about dementia's classification, about how the brain works, takes us to the center of the evolution of neuroscience.

Part of the battle over dementia's definition was whether it belonged to psychiatry or neurology, and over what that meant. In 1900, people with dementia often ended up in mental hospitals. The scientists who studied them, to the extent dementia was studied, were largely psychiatrists. The rediscovery of dementia challenged that tradition. Robert Katzman dismissed with withering disdain any connection between dementia and mental illnesses like depression. Katzman and colleagues viewed dementia as a different sort of disease, one caused by measurable brain changes, reflecting pathology that might be seen with advanced scientific imaging. That meant dementia should belong not to psychiatry, but neurology. The debate over which diseases belonged to either psychiatry or neurology was not new, but came to a head, so to speak, as twentieth century science progressed.

Starting in the nineteenth century, brain illnesses were sometimes divided into *organic* and *functional disorders. Organic* meant that doctors had figured out a plausible biological basis. *Functional* was harder to define, but the gist was that doctors couldn't pinpoint a physical pathology for a person's symptoms, so they had to be due to mental causes, meaning nonbiological psychological factors. To a first approximation, brain diseases whose biologic (or organic) basis was clear migrated to neurology. When the biological mechanism behind a disease remained more elusive, it stayed with psychiatry. Over time and in some contexts, the word *functional* took on a pejorative character—a medical form of blaming the victim. In this negative sense, *functional* meant something like "you complain, you are a mess, but I can't find a thing wrong with you. Can't be my fault. Must be yours."

Consider epilepsy. Epilepsy was once viewed as a mental illness, and a terribly stigmatized one at that. Not only were epileptics confined in mental hospitals, but even there they were denigrated. In the 1920s, there was still serious debate as to whether epilepsy was functional or organic, with some scholarly works holding fast to the functional interpretation.[1] As science discovered more about how the brain works, epilepsy was understood to be organic, not functional, and moved over to neurology. Depression and schizophrenia fell into the functional category in the nineteenth and first half of the twentieth century; scientists at that time could not identify any specific biological pathology associated with these illnesses. But careful here. Just because scientists couldn't see the biological mechanisms behind depression doesn't mean they are not there.

I am reminded of playing hide-and-seek with my daughter when she was a toddler. She would hide ineffectively, the toe of her pink sneaker sticking out from under the curtain. For good measure, she would often close her eyes. A toddler with boing-boing curls is endearing when she decides that something she can't see just can't be seen at all. But to assume that a biological mechanism for an illness doesn't exist because it can't yet be seen is less endearing in a group of scientists. Yet this was essentially the assumption behind classifying mental illnesses as functional.

The distinction between organic and functional diseases fades with time as scientists learn more about how the brain works. Many brain diseases produce symptoms on both sides of the blurry line we think of as dividing psychiatry and neurology. If you have Parkinson's disease, in addition to tremors, you have a high likelihood of depression. If you have depression, you are very likely to have abnormalities in learning and memory, and even in how you move. Current neuroscience demonstrates that all mental processes, either in health or illness, reflect physical events in the brain. When a person experiences the hallucinations of psychosis, the seizures of epilepsy, or the delight of laughing together with friends, all these experiences depend on the firing of neurons in the brain and the transmission of signals from one neuron to another through the brain's networks.[2] And when a person has a brain illness, whether it is epilepsy, dementia, or depression, some aspect of the normal functioning of the brain has gone awry. While we understand more and more about neural function, we are far from knowing all we need to know.

In the middle of the twentieth century, the division between organic and functional illnesses still meant something. The psychoanalytic viewpoint was enormously powerful and posited that psychiatric illnesses primarily result from the interplay of psychological forces and human relationships. They didn't deny the existence of biological factors and genetics, not exactly, but these were not a focus of treatment and research. Psychiatry for the most part accepted the distinction. Analytically oriented treatment explored psychological forces through conversation and memory, addressing feelings and reactions to improve function. To the psychoanalyst, mental illness was quite "real," even if it did not have identifiable physiological correlates.[3]

Other physicians disagreed. Psychiatrist Thomas Szasz was the major proponent of the view that mental illness lacked a biological basis and was merely a "myth."[4] Szasz claimed that what looked like mental illness was simply the operation of societal prejudice. He was correct that stigma has a huge impact on patients with mental illness and that psychiatry had at times failed to combat it. But on balance, Szasz's arguments have melted away as science progressed. Vast amounts of evidence now prove him wrong. Genetic links to major mental illnesses, including schizophrenia, manic depression, and depression, are well documented and are the subject of vigorous ongoing research. Szasz also claimed that no function was impaired by mental illness. It is hard to accept that such a statement could be made by someone who graduated from medical school or had ever met a seriously depressed, manic, or psychotic person. Certainly Thomas Kirkbride and Benjamin Rush recognized both the suffering and serious impairment of their nineteenth-century patients. Severe mental illness can prevent a person from working, parenting, or even eating or getting out of bed. These are not only illnesses, but illnesses that kill. It's hard to get more real than that.

But here is the tricky part. Yes, all brain illnesses have a biological basis. *And* experience, including human relationships, and the environment play a role. When bad (or good) things happen to you, they are encoded in the brain by your firing neurons. When a person endures chronic psychological abuse, it changes the brain. Actual physical neurons form networks that record the abuse. Post-traumatic stress disorder, or PTSD, can result. An abuser need never physically touch a victim's head to change and essentially damage his or her brain. The results are harder to see than those from a blow by a blunt object, but they are no less devastating. A terrifying experience triggers activity in a part of the brain known as the amygdala, which plays a role in fight-or-flight responses. The amygdala sends signals that become a memory, processed by the hippocampus. If a victim is threatened again, perhaps not by the original abuser but by someone or something that recalls the experience, that memory is triggered, and the prefrontal cortex urges a flight to safety.[5]

Your brain refuses to choose sides in the nature/nurture debate. It takes a "yes and" approach. Do genes have an impact on dementia? Yes, *and* so does your life experience, including social determinants of health like diet, fitness, and education. The good news is that many types of intervention can help with different illnesses. Medications can and do work. So too can psychotherapy and cognitive therapy, which operate by rewiring brain circuits through learning. The best treatment, as defined by solid evidence, varies with the illness and its symptoms. Indeed, the VA has released guidelines noting that current evidence supports cognitive therapy as more effective than medication in the treatment of PTSD.[6] That's not to say that all treatments are equal, nor are all brain diseases. As our classification schemes improve, we get better at gathering evidence to show what interventions work for what problems.

In the 1970s, it wasn't only psychiatrists upholding the functional/organic divide. Scientific luminary Robert Katzman scorned the notion that "functional psychiatric conditions" had any relationship to dementia.[7] He dismissed much prior work on the topic as exhibiting "intellectual disarray" because it failed to establish clear connections between neuropathology and symptoms.[8] Katzman's criticism is harsh, given that the mysterious nonlinear relationship between neuropathology and symptoms remains a central challenge in understanding dementia. Katzman and his contemporaries, brilliant though they were, were wrong in thinking that depression was "functional," and wrong that it had no connection to dementia. Today we see many connections between the two diseases, though the extent to which one is a risk factor for the other remains a topic of study.[9] Perhaps Katzman and his colleagues needed to throw over the received wisdom in order to start again. Historian Jesse Ballenger has argued compellingly that Katzman's generation owed more than they acknowledged to scholars in the mid-twentieth century.[10] Today, different scholars focus on neuroscience, big epidemiological data sets, or other approaches as they prefer, but there is widespread agreement that disparate factors like genetic risks, diet, and education all play a role in promoting or hindering the development of dementia in older people.

Bottom line: There is no clear-cut difference between mental illnesses and neurological ones. There is only one organ in your skull. These are all brain illnesses arising from critical combinations of factors, including genes and life experience. Psychiatrists and neurologists treat different illnesses, and often different symptoms of the same illnesses, in part for historical reasons, not because one type of illness is biological and one is not.

Back in the 1970s and 1980s, and even to this day, advocates proclaimed that Alzheimer's was not a mental illness. What did that mean? What was their goal? One concern was practical. Insurance did not cover mental illnesses to the same extent it covered neurological ones. For a loved one with Alzheimer's, insurance coverage in the 1980s might vanish if the disease was listed as a psychiatric disorder. One way to get fair coverage was to insist that dementia was physical, not mental. A better solution is to argue that there is no justification for insuring mental illnesses and their associated disability at a different level from other disabilities. The movement for parity in coverage for mental illness has been an important voice for social justice. Its success has to some extent extinguished the claim that dementia is not a mental illness. But you do still hear such statements from time to time, including from the Alzheimer's Association, which ought to know better.[11]

Some tried to disassociate dementia from mental illness. Rather than take the high road and fight the stigma against all illnesses with behavioral and cognitive symptoms, they insisted that dementia had nothing to do with those crazy people. It is as if Alzheimer's is an older kid on the playground, trying to ignore a disabled little brother. But at the end of the day, the family resemblance is unmistakable. Dementia is a brain illness. And so are depression and schizophrenia. The symptoms that make dementia problematic for caregivers, and embarrass or isolate those suffering with dementia, are often the same ones that lead to stigma against patients with a mental illness like schizophrenia. All should be met with compassion, not censure.

When neuroscientists in the seventies argued that dementia was not a mental illness, symptoms like agitation, depression, and psychosis were relegated to the sidelines. If only people with dementia could set aside these symptoms so easily—they include the behaviors that may get you kicked out of assisted living. There remains some bickering between psychiatry and neurology about which ought to be the primary home for dementia; this debate is not helpful to patients and caregivers. We don't need to barricade study and treatment within one medical specialty or another. We need to do just the opposite. We need to bring all relevant expertise together to work out how the brain produces symptoms and find ways to address them.

That collaboration is finally under way; important work from different fields is widely recognized. We have a lot of ground to cover. We still don't know enough about what causes or prevents dementia. We haven't done a good enough job of disseminating to clinicians what we *do* know about managing symptoms and preserving cognitive function. But all experts agree that dementia is a brain disease, one in which cells in the brain fail and die. When Jonathan Swift said he would die at the top, this was not just a metaphor. The neurons of the brain die in dementia.

The second barrier to research progress is the Darwinian struggle for funding. In the 1970s, Lewis Thomas called Alzheimer's "the disease of the century."[12] Brilliant though he was, he spoke too soon. If we speak of the impact of a disease in terms of both terror and funding, we should speak of the elephant in the room, one that was unknown when Thomas made his comment. That elephant is not Alzheimer's; it is AIDS. AIDS was the disease of the twentieth century, or at least its last quarter.

AIDS, like Alzheimer's, started out obscure. AIDS first appears, though not by name, in the June 1981 weekly report of the Centers for Disease Control and Prevention (CDC), briefly summarizing five cases of young men who died of a rare pneumonia. By the turn of the millennium, AIDS was the fourth most common cause of death *globally,* and by far the most common cause in sub-Saharan Africa.[13] The meteoric crash with which AIDS entered the public consciousness, the staggering early mortality rates, the misinformation spread far and wide, and the shameful behavior, often from medical professionals, toward those afflicted by the illness were beyond compare. Yet quickly enough—by bureaucratic standards, at least—the increase in funding for research and the extraordinary speed of scientific progress regarding AIDS outstripped that of other diseases of the twentieth century. The first federal funding specifically for AIDS was passed in 1983, with $12 million. By 1985—*two years later*—Congress had allocated $190 million for AIDS research, tens of millions more than requested.[14] In that year, Alzheimer's funding also rose, but only to $53 million. By 1989, the CDC estimated that AIDS had hit 100,000 patients in the United States.[15] About 1 million Americans had Alzheimer's.[16] By any count, research spending per person with HIV/AIDS, then and now, greatly exceeds that for each person with Alzheimer's. For the roughly 1 million patients in the U.S. with HIV/AIDS today, compared with the 5 million patients with dementia, per capita spending is about ten times more—and that includes dramatic increases in dementia research in the last few years.[17] Various expert panels on dementia have estimated that it would take $2 billion a year to move the dial substantially toward finding effective treatments. (That's about the level of domestic AIDS research funding.) As of this writing, dementia receives a bit above $1 billion per year, after several substantial yearly increases under President Obama. The Trump administration initially proposed whopping cuts to NIH funding. However, bipartisan congressional support, plus major efforts from the Alzheimer's Association and allies, secured an additional $400 million in funding for Alzheimer's research in 2017.[18]

To be very clear, I do not favor spending less on AIDS research or treatment. My training as a doctor was profoundly shaped by the AIDS crisis. I treated many young people with AIDS, many of whom died, badly and too soon. AIDS is not for me an abstract problem. My internship came at the height of the crisis, and just before the advent of regulations limiting hours for doctors in training to an average of eighty hours a week. For me, that year revolved around two themes: sleep deprivation and AIDS. I recall one man my age and, like me, a lapsed Irish Catholic. He was a mortally ill, blue-eyed rogue who looked like the dark Irish boys I grew up with. He was frightened. We had little to offer him. We gave him antibiotics to treat his pneumonia, but that was just a Band-Aid. He got out of the hospital and I lost track of him. Most likely he died before I finished my medical training. I don't ever want us to go back to that state of ignorance. Research funding made the difference, largely due to AIDS activism. That, and massive efforts at education, which focused not only on treatment and testing but also on teaching people how safer sex and clean needles could slow the rate of infection.

In the 1980s and since, most proponents for additional funds for Alzheimer's research were careful to tread lightly around the topic of

AIDS. They wanted more funding for Alzheimer's, not less for AIDS. That creates a delicate balance, of course, since even the largesse of the federal government has limits. There cannot be more funding for every disease. Most advocates pushed for their own cause without attacking others. One exception was Jesse Helms, who once stood up in the Senate and demanded reduced AIDS funding to give more money to deserving victims of Alzheimer's. Alzheimer's advocates strongly objected.[19]

However, in subtle ways the comparison did infiltrate the debate about how to allocate scarce research funds. A *Congressional Quarterly* report from the 1980s describes Alzheimer's as "a mysterious disease because it doesn't discriminate between its victims—there is no pattern to the race, sex, or lifestyle of those it strikes."[20] Today's better epidemiological information proves the statement false—there *are* differences in rates of dementia across race and ethnicity, gender, and lifestyle. But more important, the description invites comparison to another prominent disease, one tightly linked to gay men, whose "lifestyle factors" carried an enormous burden of stigma. Helms was not alone in drawing attention to the "innocence" of victims of Alzheimer's, in contrast to those with AIDS.

The example of AIDS is useful for more than pointing out the challenge of competing against worthy recipients for research funds. AIDS treatment gives us one idea of what progress can look like. That knowledge will be useful as we turn to the third and most difficult challenge of dementia research: actually solving the scientific problem. For AIDS, we now have effective medicines that must be taken for a person's lifetime. There have been important pushes to make them affordable both domestically and in developing countries, and these have had a momentous impact in increasing life expectancy and quality of life for those with HIV/AIDS. Programs that address high-risk behaviors are also crucial; condoms and needle exchange programs have helped decrease exposure. Today, AIDS can be managed as a chronic illness. That is a huge success, on par with the fight against polio. But with polio we found an effective prevention in a vaccine. We do not have a cure for AIDS.

So is AIDS the model of success for dementia? Lewis Thomas once wrote that the most important forms of medical technology are those that cure or prevent disease.[21] He labeled as less desirable what he called "halfway technology," those interventions that merely support or maintain function without curing the underlying illness. Thomas lived in the optimistic generation of physicians who believed you just had to find an infecting agent and cure it with an antibiotic or prevent it with a vaccine. AIDS took us down a peg. It showed us we were not nearly as smart as we thought we were. We've learned that viruses can be fiendishly clever and change their structure, thwarting efforts to create a vaccine. Bacteria have adapted to the point that many are no longer susceptible to our arsenal of antibiotics. We made it easy for them by feeding antibiotics wantonly to farmyard animals and handing them out like Halloween candy for viral illnesses like colds where they have no impact. This has slashed our chances of conquering bacteria; they've seen all our weapons and know how to fight back. AIDS provides a distinct vision for what success looks like. It also reaffirms the need for clinical humility in medicine.

That humility is further supported by the nature of medicine's gains against illnesses like diabetes and heart disease. Physicians generally do not think of cure as the norm anymore. Most major illnesses are chronic. We would like to cure, but we don't expect to. We manage. We try to convert an illness that can kill you into one you can live with, one that won't kill you so quickly. For heart disease we try one or several medicines, stop others, and encourage changes in behavior and diet. Smoking makes most chronic illnesses worse, so we urge patients to quit. That is how doctors today approach heart disease, diabetes, lung disease, even many cancers.

That's where medicine has arrived, in the twenty-first century. We don't expect a slam dunk. We look for interventions that delay symptoms and make them more manageable. That approach has brought great success in battling the illnesses of the twenty-first century. These diseases are still killers, but we can often delay death. That's no small thing. Some more quality years with your family look pretty sweet when you thought you were headed out the door. We live longer, with disability. What we ought to be looking for are the tools to manage dementia, to slow it down. You'll notice I don't say cure. When we ask for research funding, we have to articulate how we're going to tackle the problem. Looking for a cure is not the same as looking to manage dementia.

My reluctance to pound the drum for cure will get me in trouble with good people who are working hard to combat Alzheimer's. The federal government's committee for Alzheimer's policy, the National Alzheimer's Project Act (NAPA), initially called for a cure by 2020.[22] Not going to happen. Sorry. They now have a more reasonable statement on their website, calling for effective treatment by 2025. That's still a stretch, but a more plausible one. It's not that I take dementia lightly. I am pretty sure it's heading my way. But a plan that's likely to fail, that is not based on feasible goals, is not a useful one, and it can delay progress toward one that might actually get us closer.

That brings us to the third major barrier, the challenge of just doing science. Scientists set out to define the problem of Alzheimer's and get funding, and then went to work on solving the puzzle before them. Science is hard. A thousand theories bloomed. Researchers rushed to find a cause, investigating toxic agents, infections, genetics, whatever they could think of. Early on, some researchers found high levels of aluminum in the postmortem brains of those with Alzheimer's, and thus was born the theory that Alzheimer's was a reaction to excess aluminum. This theory grabbed the popular imagination, especially after it was linked to acid rain, a newly identified environmental threat resulting from air pollution. For a time, anxious buyers shunned aluminum pans.[23] Sober minds ultimately prevailed, pointing out that aluminum is among the most ubiquitous substances on earth, and it is in the brains of those with and without dementia. So scratch that idea off the list.

Many scientists wondered if a virus was the cause of Alzheimer's. In the 1980s, researchers were unlocking basic viral mechanisms and finding connections to cancers, hepatitis, and AIDs. Intriguingly, an unusual form of dementia called kuru was found to be transmitted by a virus, one that tribesmen in eastern New Guinea acquired by eating the brains of deceased infected people. Though brain-eating remains, erm, uncommon, this finding showed that viruses *could* cause dementia. Maybe a slow virus, one that slumbers for years before symptoms emerge, would be the source. Many looked; no one found. These paths did not produce credible evidence linking Alzheimer's to a toxin or a virus.

That is not to say these theories died out instantly and altogether. There are always those who cling to a belief after the scientific mainstream has abandoned it. Put differently, the mainstream may reject evidence that a minority finds convincing. Science has awarded victories to those in both camps. Many great thinkers, Einstein among them, were originally ridiculed by peers who could not grasp the weight of a new theory or new evidence. Sometimes the lone voice is correct. Just not very often. (The ratio of Einsteins to people who are simply wrong has always been low.)

Mostly, the majority of people with expertise in a field get it right, at least in time. They want to succeed and follow what look like the best clues. They set aside approaches that don't pan out, though this can be hard once one has invested a lot of time, effort, and personal reputation in a particular pathway. It may take a while to turn away from those rusty old approaches, but over time the path that solves problems and brings results is the one that acquires adherents. This phenomenon of progress in science was most famously described by Thomas Kuhn in *The Structure of Scientific Revolutions*.[24] If you are a baby boomer and graduated from college, it's likely you read this book; it showed up in several of my undergraduate courses. Kuhn investigates how science moves from one overarching theory to another. As part of that, he addresses how scientists deal with theories and facts that annoyingly fail to fit in with scientific evidence. Often, scientists can show that what looks like a contradiction is just wrong data or a wrong interpretation. This is what happened with the theory of aluminum as a causal agent for Alzheimer's; better studies undermined the early claims, and the field moved on in its search for a cause, although there were a few holdouts for a while longer.

It wasn't hard to disprove. The contraindications to aluminum as a cause came in early, so there was no set of powerful institutions that had made their living off the aluminum theory, and few oxen were gored when the field moved on. But crossing a scientific theory off the list gets exponentially harder when careers and dollars and institutional reputations are at stake. Then you see adherents man the barricades, doing all they can to prop up a failing hypothesis. With aluminum, the system worked. An interesting theory was followed up, checked out by diverse researchers, and then set aside in the absence of sound supporting evidence. Unfortunately, Alzheimer's research has not always followed this pattern.

Sometimes, evidence is unclear or conflicting about whether a given factor plays a role in disease development. For instance, some early researchers wondered if Alzheimer's was a form of autoimmune disease, in which the body attacks itself. Perhaps the body was attacking the abnormal proteins that make up the characteristic plaques and tangles, and the results of that attack caused symptoms. Researchers did find some evidence in the brains of Alzheimer's patients to support this theory.[25] Or perhaps those plaques and tangle were the body's attempt to protect itself from attack by something else. Current research has unearthed immune responses that unleash neurochemicals causing inflammation, accelerating the pathologic process of Alzheimer's.[26] There have long been and still are many investigators of the immunology of dementia. They have unearthed many clues, but still no cure.

One early success was what became known as the cholinergic hypothesis. Three articles in the 1970s from three different labs suggested it, nearly simultaneously, with varying degrees of clarity. The earliest and longest paper of the three addresses the tribulations of measuring neurotransmitters in the brain after death; measurements get muddier as time passes and the body breaks down. It notes, almost in passing, that levels of an enzyme related to the neurotransmitter acetylcholine are lower in Alzheimer's disease, suggesting that the related cholinergic system might be involved in memory deficits.[27] (Cholinergic means, more or less, related to acetylcholine, an important chemical in brain function.) But this suggestion is buried within a good deal of other substantive work.

A clearer statement comes in a brief letter to the editor of *The Lancet* in 1976 by Peter Davies and A. J. F. Maloney, both in Edinburgh at that time.[28] They had the happy thought to test the activity of different neurotransmitters in the postmortem brains of those with Alzheimer's and those without. Levels of two enzymes required to create

acetylcholine were greatly reduced in the brains of those with Alzheimer's. Intriguingly, exactly the areas that showed reductions in
these enzymes were those with the most neurofibrillary tangles. The
authors argue that Alzheimer's pathology includes a specific reduction
in the cholinergic system in the cortex. This brief letter was thrilling
to the elite cadre of Alzheimer's researchers—this was something gen-
uinely new.[29]

The final of the three publications, also a brief, career-making letter
in *The Lancet,* appeared only a month later, and draws connections yet
more explicitly. Elaine Perry and her colleagues note that the dopamine
deficit in Parkinson's disease can be "countered, with clinical benefit,"
by supplementing the dopamine system. They report their observations
on low levels of cholinergic substances in senile dementia, and call for
research seeking therapeutic interventions that will supplement exactly
this deficit.[30] The cholinergic hypothesis was born. Simply stated, it
runs thus: Brains with Alzheimer's have too little of cholinergic neurotransmitters, and therapy could try to overcome that deficit.

Immediately, many groups set out to work on the cholinergic hypothesis. Before the year was out, a publication showed a glimmer of
promise by enhancing cholinergic substances in Alzheimer's.[31] True,
gains were very modest indeed—they did not show up on standard
cognitive measures—but the idea remained promising. A few years
later, Peter Whitehouse's team at Johns Hopkins made a crucial discovery by locating an area where cholinergic neurons were gravely de-
pleted in Alzheimer's patients.[32] This tiny patch of brain has a big
name: the nucleus basalis of Meynert. It normally makes cholinergic
substances and projects them to the cortex. Examination of this area
in the brain of an Alzheimer's patient showed a radical decrease as
compared with a control patient, and gave scientists a specific location
for the deficit suggested by the cholinergic hypothesis.

By 1986, W. K. Summers and his colleagues published in *The New England Journal of Medicine* a small study showing improvement in patients using tacrine, the drug that would become the first FDA-approved medication for Alzheimer's dementia.[33] Researchers often crow about exciting findings, or come as close as a staid scientific journal will permit. Here, however, the authors modestly describe tacrine only as a possible palliative treatment. An accompanying editorial by researchers not involved in the study acknowledges their achievement, but also casts serious shade. They note, "Any therapeutic strategy that relies on the integrity of the cholinergic neuron for its efficacy in a degenerative brain condition like Alzheimer's disease is ultimately flawed."[34] To translate, there is an obvious problem with tacrine: It can't cure Alzheimer's. Tacrine slows down the process that breaks down acetylcholine, so it sticks around longer in the brain. It does not, however, actually supply more acetylcholine. It relies on the brain to do that, despite the fact that as Alzheimer's progresses, the brain loses the ability to create acetylcholine. There will come a time when this strategy must fail, and in fact the most severely affected patients in the small study received little benefit. Worse still, it was already possible to say, as that early editorial did, that Alzheimer's involved deficits in multiple neurotransmitters, not just in cholinergic ones. There were limits to the possible success of cholinergic agents, and they were visible before the first drug was ever approved.[35]

Tacrine was approved for treating Alzheimer's in 1993. Additional drugs that amped up the cholinergic system followed, with donepezil in 1996 and galantamine in 2001. These drugs are palliative, just as that early article on tacrine noted. They help decrease some symptoms in some people for some time, generally months, not years.[36] They are not a cure, and no cure will come from a better drug based on this mechanism. One other drug, memantine, also with limited efficacy, was the most recently approved in the United States, in 2003. That's it for dementia drugs—countless millions of dollars, three decades of continuing research, and no victory in finding a drug that changes the course of Alzheimer's disease.

Dementia specialists have different opinions about the benefits of this class of drugs. Joe Verghese is professor of Neurology and Chief of the Division of Geriatrics at Montefiore Health System. He is a dementia expert and dedicated clinician who takes a modestly positive view, finding that a subset of patients benefit dramatically, at least for a time. The improvement may not show up on standard tests of cognitive function, but families report that their relative participates in activities, including conversations, in a way that has not been possible for years.[37] Other clinicians are more negative, and see these medicines as essentially expensive placebos whose main effect is to enrich pharmaceutical companies—particularly galling when medications are ineffective. Stopping these medicines may be challenging, partly because families are so desperate to see improvements. These drugs, despite their limitations, are the only game in town. They are widely prescribed, often in combinations and for years. It is hard for doctors to say, and for patients and families to hear, that we do not have a medication that can change the course of Alzheimer's disease. That's where we are now. That's all we've got.

There has been enormous progress toward the goal of understanding how brain processes break down to produce dementia. Yet we still contend with all three of these barriers. We still struggle to define the problem of dementia in a way that promotes real progress. There will always be a struggle for funding. And the battle to solve the scientific puzzle rages on.

Chapter 8

The Amyloid Hypothesis Falls Apart

W e have failed to find effective treatments or prevention for dementia, despite years of searching by some of the world's best scientists. Is this a tragedy? Let's see: A classical tragedy demands several elements. The story must arouse pity and fear. You need a hero, one whose misfortunes arise not from vice and depravity, but from errors of judgment and frailty.

Stories about science are often framed as heroic narratives, in which a lonely scientist triumphs. For the most part, that story is bullshit. That's not how science works, not today and mostly not ever. Scientists may or may not be lonely, and some stay up late by themselves in the lab, but they do not work in isolation. Multimillion-dollar grants do not go to the modern-day Madame Curie, soldiering on in the irradiated gloom. They go to dozens, sometimes thousands of researchers, in a slew of collaborating institutions. And it's hard to know, in real time, what's an error in judgment and what is a promising pathway that doesn't pay off. We love the idea of the eureka moment—problem solved. But the way science moves forward is not generally through the knockout punch. Success comes more often as a little girlish slap in the face of the unknown. Incrementally, those tiny pats constitute progress. Stories of epic wins are written after the fact, and leave out all the missteps, the errors in judgment. They sell well. Alas, they are not true. We are still in the middle of the scientific story of dementia. We are not at a triumphal moment, but neither could you call the story a tragedy.

In elite institutions around the world, brilliant men and women rack their tip-top brains working on dementia. These people are astonishing. Just to list their achievements takes dozens of pages, chock-full of references to Harvard, Oxford, and the National Academy of Sciences. They win prestigious prizes and millions in grant funding. Every one of those researchers faces the painful knowledge that there is no cure. There is no cure today, and not likely in time for the generation of baby boomers. That arouses pity and fear in me, and should in the rest of us who are middle-aged or more. The lack of a cure is tragic for those who need one today. But science plays the long game. We can't simply order a cure for what ails us. Science works on the problems it can reach with today's knowledge. I try not to take it personally. Even with all that pity and fear, really, this is just science, just the way it works.

The search for new drugs for dementia has been brutally difficult. Drug trials for treatments have an unusually low success rate, far worse than for cancer drugs. Efforts to find new medications for dementia have a 99.6 percent failure rate.[1] That's appalling. And even if researchers discover something that works, it can take twelve years to go from inspiration through FDA-approved trials to market. We might decrease this time lag by revising regulations, but we can't eliminate it altogether; whenever you speed up the review process, you increase the chance of rushing a risky drug to market.

But here's an even bigger problem: The brain changes that lead to dementia begin years before symptoms start, maybe decades. Many scientists believe that prevention—before brain damage occurs—is the best way to beat dementia. A lot of today's research is aimed at those who have no symptoms or are barely affected. While early interventions may help reduce dementia long-term, they can do nothing for those who already have moderate or severe disease. The brunt of our efforts has effectively written off those who are already ill. We have millions with dementia now, and will keep adding millions for years to come. That's not speculation. As with the sinking *Titanic,* it is a mathematical certainty.

What a bummer. You may react by recalling headlines trumpeting great research that brings us to the brink of cure. Perhaps you are thinking of verubecestat, celebrated in an article titled "Alzheimer's Treatment Within Reach After Successful Drug Trial."[2] This drug passed a Phase 1 trial in November 2016, avoiding the pitfall of serious liver toxicity that killed earlier similar agents. Here is where I, in my role as Debbie Downer, MD, must remind you that 99.6 percent of experimental drugs to treat Alzheimer's fail. Of those that get through Phase 1, which addresses safety but not efficacy, 98 percent fail. That was verubecestat's big achievement: it reached a 98 percent probability of failure. It also showed some worrisome safety issues. By February 2017, Merck shut down the Phase 3 trial in those with mild to moderate dementia. They tried a new study for those with very early symptoms, which was a dismal failure; the group receiving medicine had more side effects and slightly worse cognitive outcomes.[3] Verubecestat fell by the wayside, just like many of its competitors. Of the 244 compounds assessed from 2002 to 2012, exactly one made it to market: memantine, which does not attack the underlying mechanism of disease.

Or maybe you saw the story on *60 Minutes* concerning a drug trial going on in remote Colombia?[4] That study focuses on a small isolated cohort with genetically determined early onset dementia. The current trial ($100 million, financed jointly by Genentech and NIA) is using a drug called crenezumab. They hope that giving the drug in the earliest possible phase—before people with the abnormal gene have symptoms—will prevent dementia. I hope they're right. In my role as killjoy, however, I note that crenezumab already failed Phase 2 trials for those with mild to moderate symptoms.[5] That failure doesn't let us foresee the future, but it's not a great sign.

Is there another drug now in trials that could pass this gauntlet? I don't believe so. I hope I'm wrong. A lot of the current crop have already failed significant trials or are similar to medications that have. Some of the hype you see may reflect the triumph of hope over experience. That's easy to understand: Everyone would like a cure! Then again, even a so-so Alzheimer's drug can make a lot of money, because there's nothing better out there. So that hype may also reflect excitement about profit rather than progress.

Triumphal stories vastly outnumber stories about how those same drugs don't pan out. Journalists would rather write and we would rather read stories headlined: "Ta-da! Here comes the cure." There's no fun in "No cure coming. We're going to have to keep taking care of people with this chronic illness." But that's the true story, and the false narrative of cure puts us seriously off course. Don't misunderstand me: We need to keep working on the scientific puzzle of dementia. We also need to sober up. This problem is not going away. When we focus excessively on cure, we undermine care.

Many dementia researchers have a deep personal stake in the outcome of their work. Scholar after scholar told me of a parent with dementia. Reisa Sperling, director of the Center for Alzheimer Research and Treatment at Harvard Medical School and one of the world's great experts in the field, has both a grandfather and a father with dementia. Sperling is a warm, concerned physician-researcher who aims her impressive bandwidth at the scientific challenge of dementia. She knows better than anyone the cost of delay in making better treatments, and that once symptoms are present it may be too late to help. She noted, "My dad unfortunately has mild AD (Alzheimer's disease), and I worry about what can be done for him. As a clinical neurologist, when I see people in my office that have mild to moderate dementia . . . unless I can get them in the clinical trial and it really works and they happen to be on the drug rather than a placebo, for them personally we have lost the battle."[6]

Sperling is right to worry. American baby boomers are turning sixty-five at the rate of 10,000 people a day. Since the pathology that causes Alzheimer's begins years before symptoms do, you can't prevent the illness unless you reach people who are in their fifties and sixties— even earlier might be better. The window is closing during which prevention can help even the youngest baby boomers. Other people may benefit in the future, but we won't have prevented dementia in millions of people who are age fifty and up today. It isn't for lack of trying, but defeats outnumber victories.

Let's examine some of those defeats and victories. Dementia research started up again in earnest in the 1970s and has gained steam ever since. Scientists have learned a great deal since then. Amyloid plaques and tau tangles precede the death of neurons, though specifics of the process are hotly debated. Amyloid and tau are not born bad; they have jobs in healthy brains but fall under malignant influences and make trouble. Amyloid's precursor protein helps move cholesterol and helps brain cells stick together in useful ways,[7] while tau helps maintain orderly tubules that keep neural cells and the brain's information highway working smoothly.[8] Amyloid's precursor protein gets cut by enzymes into various pieces, some of which result in beta-amyloid, which forms sticky plaques outside of brain cells, and also circulates in the blood in a soluble form; both are implicated in brain pathology leading to Alzheimer's dementia.[9] Tau, like other proteins, often gets tagged with molecules that switch functions on and off, but sometimes abnormal tagging proceeds to a tangled, malfunctioning form of tau.

The lion's share of research funding for the last twenty-five years has gone to research based on the amyloid hypothesis, proposed by John Hardy and David Allsop in 1991.[10] They theorized that the deposition of sticky beta-amyloid plaques initiates Alzheimer's pathology, and that leads to multiple downstream toxic changes, including chemical alterations in tau, the formation of tau tangles, and finally, the death of neural cells. The theory has had many powerful adherents and substantial supporting data. But right from the start, there have been detractors. A kind of Hatfield and McCoy battle grew between those scientists who focused on beta-amyloid plaques (BAPtists) as the main cause of Alzheimer's and those who believed that the role of tau tangles was under-recognized (Tauists). Proclamations popped up regularly over the years that this war was over, yet funding continued to flow to BAPtists at the expense of Tauists or those with yet different approaches. Now, however, the amyloid hypothesis has taken a beating; it may never recover. At a minimum, it requires substantial revision. Researchers looking at other mechanisms and pathways grapple with questions left unanswered by the amyloid hypothesis, at least in its basic form. To understand the failure to find effective new drugs for Alzheimer's, we need to retrace the rise and fall of the amyloid hypothesis.

The focus on amyloid reflects the "Alzheimerization" of dementia, which started with the successful marketing efforts of scientists, lobbyists, and the Alzheimer's Association in the 1970s and 1980s.[11] The strategy worked—dementia carved out a name for itself as a real disease, not just a normal consequence of aging. The downside was a crowding out of symptoms, contributing factors, and other forms of dementia irrelevant to Alzheimer's. Memory loss and amyloid were where the money was, literally. The facts that aging of the brain *is* implicated in dementia, that other illnesses and other forms of dementia overlap with Alzheimer's, and that symptoms like depression, agitation, psychosis, and the loss of executive function are all common in dementia were diminished in importance and in research funding. So much funding goes into studying Alzheimer's that it's easy to forget there are other types of dementia, and that millions of people suffer from them.

The amyloid hypothesis did what a good theory does: It tied together intriguing, disparate pieces of evidence. Genetic research played a big role, locating a gene crucial for making amyloid on chromosome 21. People with Down syndrome have three instead of the normal two copies of chromosome 21; that's the meaning of Down syndrome's official name, trisomy 21. They have excess amyloid and develop Alzheimer's disease at very high rates and an early age. This amyloid buildup in people with Down syndrome is a cornerstone of the amyloid hypothesis. Too much amyloid looks like it leads to Alzheimer's in Down syndrome, so that must be what happens to other Alzheimer's patients, too.

The amyloid hypothesis also relies on genetic research from a few places in the world with odd clusters of early onset dementia, like that region of Colombia highlighted in the *60 Minutes* episode. There, isolated geography and intermarriage mean that many people inherit a single mutated gene that causes dementia by age forty.[12] Around the world at least 180 different gene mutations on various chromosomes lead to autosomal dominant Alzheimer's disease (ADAD).[13]

ADAD has attracted research interest and funding out of proportion to the number of people who suffer from it. ADAD accounts for less than 1 percent of all cases of Alzheimer's. The driving force behind this research is not just to solve the problem of ADAD. Since some people with an ADAD gene have a nearly 100 percent likelihood of developing Alzheimer's, scientists can study them while they are well and track changes in their blood, memory, and brains. That information may lead to blood tests or other markers that predict dementia. Some of these highly motivated, at-risk people try experimental medicines to see if they slow or stop the development of symptoms. The hope is that a medicine will work not only in the few people with ADAD but also in the vast number of people at risk for late onset AD.

More than one dementia researcher compared this approach— looking at ADAD to solve the puzzle of late onset dementia—to the discovery of the cholesterol-lowering statin drugs.[14] A family with a rare form of inherited high cholesterol benefited from taking the first statin, and then statins turned out to work for the common non-inherited form of high cholesterol. That class of drug became one of Big Pharma's blockbusters. Researchers want to help families with the terrible scourge of early dementia, but they don't object to doing well by doing good. One reason to study ADAD is the hope of finding a miracle cure for Alzheimer's and becoming a zillionaire in the process. No one has found this pot of gold, despite lots of research dollars and fifteen years of searching.

But here is where things get complicated. Not only are there many forms of dementia, there are many forms of Alzheimer's. Those who get dementia in old age don't have a single determining gene; the illness results from multiple interacting factors, genetic and otherwise. A crude rule of thumb is that the earlier the onset of dementia is, the more likely it is that a dominant gene controls the process and the less important other factors like diet or vascular disease are. Supporters of the amyloid hypothesis argue that pathological changes in the brain in early and late onset Alzheimer's follow a similar path: Amyloid plaque accumulates, tau tangles within the neurons, and later the neurons die. This assertion—that the pathways to dementia in ADAD and late onset dementia are the same, or at least sufficiently similar—is central to the current controversy about the amyloid hypothesis. Most researchers agree that amyloid plays some role in every type of Alzheimer's. But as problems have cropped up in big research trials, more and more researchers now believe there are key differences between early and late onset dementia, enough so that a different combination of factors causes dementia in these different forms of the illness. Older brains don't make too much amyloid, for instance, but seem to have trouble getting rid of it. The field is divided on the question of how much we'll learn about late onset dementia—the kind that millions of people have—by looking at early onset dementia. At a minimum, we'll need to uncover factors specific to dementia in old age and figure out how to change them.

Richard Mayeux, chair of Neurology at Columbia University's College of Physicians and Surgeons, has a multimillion-dollar NIH grant to study rare genes associated with early onset Alzheimer's. Mayeux argues that understanding the genetics of dementia is important even if the amyloid hypothesis fades into the background, and it's hard to disagree with this.[15] I knew Mayeux thirty years ago at Columbia, and because he is of that boyish astronaut-athlete type, today he appears more or less the same, while I look like a healthy person who is thirty years older. Annoying. He does not seem to have ever exhibited a major error in judgment. In fact, pretty much everything he works on turns to gold. Mayeux has published upward of five hundred scholarly articles on an unusually broad array of topics. He believes that ADAD and late onset Alzheimer's take different paths toward dementia, and that we'll need to look at the aging brain to solve the riddle of late onset dementia. He thinks that those most likely to benefit from his research into rare ADAD genes are those with ADAD. If an intervention that helps those with ADAD also helps us understand late onset dementia, that will be fine, too. Many articles about dementia research and about Mayeux take a triumphal tone. He does not. Neither Mayeux nor the other scientists I interviewed have found a cure, but they are not tragic heroes, either. They are moving science forward.

Genes do play a role in late onset dementia, but a more nuanced and complex one than in ADAD. More than twenty gene mutations are linked to late onset AD, but none has the slam-dunk power found in the early onset form.[16] The most common of these influencing genes is known as APOE e4, which has functions related to cholesterol and amyloid. Many people without APOE e4 develop dementia. However, having one copy of this gene increases the risk of Alzheimer's by about three times and lowers the age of onset; having two—one from each parent—increases risk by fifteen times and lowers the age of onset even more.[17] In contrast, the APOE e2 variant protects against dementia and delays the age of onset.[18] That's the gene you want, but you don't get to pick your parents. Still, knowing a person has two copies of that risky APOE e4 is a far cry from knowing when and even if he will develop Alzheimer's. One study uncovered a test subject with two copies of the APOE e4 gene, over the age of a hundred, without dementia.[19] To reiterate, this person had a double dose of the best known genetic risk factor for late onset dementia, and made it to a hundred without the disease. Risk factors are not the same as a diagnosis! While you shouldn't count on being that lucky centenarian, this study underscores that there is a big difference between being at risk and being sure you will develop a disease.

Despite its dominance in research efforts, the amyloid hypothesis is under siege. A large number of clinical trials have tried to reduce or delay symptoms of dementia by reducing amyloid. These trials have failed. Some of the largest were spectacular and very expensive failures. They generated a lot of controversy among researchers, and a lot of hand-wringing at NIH and in the pharmaceutical industry. Lots of effort, time, and research dollars, but no benefit for participants.

Let's look at two large clinical trials, among the many that have failed over the last two decades. Despite constituting a who's who of dementia research, they belly flopped into *The New England Journal of Medicine* in 2014.[20] One pair of studies used a drug called bapineuzumab to try lowering amyloid in those with and without the risk-elevating APOE e4 gene.[21] The studies took place over eighteen months with thousands of participants at two hundred research sites. Those who got the active drug, not the placebo, had side effects that got worse as the dose got bigger, and included brain swelling. Though promising in earlier trials, bapineuzumab failed to improve clinical outcomes. So here's the score: side effects, but no clinical benefit.

The second set of trials involved the drug solanezumab, or sola for short. Two thousand participants with mild to moderate dementia, eighteen months, hundreds of sites, and no evidence of statistically significant clinical improvement.[22] And that remains the key problem with the amyloid hypothesis. We can reduce amyloid, but it hasn't made people better.

Intriguingly, with careful sifting through the data, it turns out that not everyone in the trials had Alzheimer's disease. The research participants were referred by specialists and all had typical symptoms. But for patients to meet the scientific definition, they must have excess amyloid plaques in their brain. Until recent years amyloid could not be seen in living people and was detected only on autopsy. All that changed with the advent of a special form of PET scan that reveals amyloid in living people. It turns out that 25 percent or more of the participants had negative scans—they didn't have enough amyloid plaque for an official diagnosis.[23] They had the symptoms, but didn't have the right pathology. No wonder lowering amyloid didn't help these patients—they didn't have an amyloid problem. If you looked at the data of people who did have amyloid plaques and very mild disease, the results looked a bit better. So maybe one reason the trials failed is that lots of participants didn't actually have the condition being studied and so failed to improve with a treatment for that condition. But skeptical scientist Michael Gold points out that the participants with normal amyloid should have been randomly distributed between the placebo and active drug groups. It shouldn't have made any difference in the trial's outcome.[24]

The implications of this discovery—that we've been overdiagnosing Alzheimer's—are far bigger than a problem with a few research studies. This means that even specialists can't predict who has Alzheimer's based on clinical symptoms. We tell people they have Alzheimer's disease; what they have is dementia. We prescribe medicine on the assumption that they all have Alzheimer's disease, but in about a fourth to a third of the cases, we're wrong. Should clinicians keep prescribing the same medicines to patients who may not have Alzheimer's disease? We don't yet know the answer to that question. We don't know which medicines, if any, help them. The amyloid focus has created a big gap for this large group of people with dementia but no amyloid problem. We need to get busy thinking about who they are, what causes their dementia, and how we can help them.

Pro-amyloid researchers argue that the main reason for the poor results in these trials was that the intervention came too late. They argue that once amyloid has piled up around your neurons and gummed up the works, cells may be irreversibly damaged and there is no turning back. This is not an outlandish position—if you want to keep someone's kidney healthy, you don't wait until he has end-stage kidney damage to try to turn things around. A much better idea is to prevent damage before it happens.

This theory—that the idea of reducing amyloid was right but the timing was wrong—holds enormous sway among amyloid proponents. The push for ever-earlier intervention has been the thread that unites all current amyloid-based clinical trials, even before the 2014 failures of sola and bapineuzumab. The amyloid hypothesis was under intense scrutiny, for a decade had gone by without a new medication for dementia, and failed trials were piling up. Skeptics multiplied, even while pro-amyloid researchers held major sway over funding decisions at NIH and in the pharmaceutical industry. Everyone agreed that efforts to reduce amyloid and improve symptoms in people with dementia had been disappointing. By then, it was clear that brain changes related to dementia began years before symptoms appeared. Proponents of the amyloid hypothesis latched onto the possibility that they had the right intervention but the wrong timing. They would try to reduce or prevent amyloid accumulation before it ever damaged delicate brain tissues.

This focus on intervening before damage occurs shaped the 2011 revision of definitions of the stages of Alzheimer's. If scientists could identify brains at risk before symptoms formed, perhaps they could beat dementia. Thus was born a new phase of Alzheimer's: preclinical Alzheimer's disease, in which a person feels fine, has no symptoms, and yet has excess amyloid plaques. Preclinical Alzheimer's disease is an attempt to save the amyloid hypothesis. Most of these people will not develop dementia, but the group is at higher risk than the general population. These people might benefit from early intervention. But this new category also created problems, ethical ones among them.[25] The stigma of dementia is enormous. Should research subjects be informed of their status in this group? They might not ever develop dementia, and there is still no effective treatment if they do.

These ethical challenges are real, but to me are not the most troubling issue associated with preclinical Alzheimer's. Prevention sounds good, but there are lots of ways to prevent illness. We can decrease lung cancer and heart disease by stopping cigarette use. We can prevent measles through a vaccine. I am concerned about a strategy that focuses on creating a drug that must be taken daily for years to treat millions of people who are at risk but not ill. The majority of them will never become ill, and even those who develop dementia likely would not do so for years, with or without the drug. It will be impossible in the individual case to know if the drug is working. If the person stays well, we won't know if the drug worked or if this person was never heading toward dementia in the first place. Some will develop dementia, but we won't know if the drug slowed down cognitive decline, or if the person progressed as he or she would have without the drug.

Suppose we have such a drug—I'll call it BrainUp@—that could be taken by anyone over the age of fifty who is worried about dementia. This is not an idle thought experiment. It is the principal strategy toward which millions of research dollars are now pointed. I'd like to prevent dementia, but I worry about using a daily medication, as opposed to a vaccine or lifestyle changes, to do it. We won't have such a treatment soon, but I am worried about what happens if it does come to market.

Start by reflecting on the size of the windfall such a drug would be to the pharmaceutical industry. I don't think everything Big Pharma does is wrong just because they do it; I am grateful to those who have worked to bring us effective medications for AIDS and cancer, and Big Pharma deserves credit as part of that success. But there are more than 75 million baby boomers who might be eligible for BrainUp@. Even if we limit access to those with an elevated risk via excess amyloid and/or an APOE e4 gene, the potential to make money is vast. This could be the mother of all blockbusters. The allure is strong, and in part stems from a potentially humongous pot of gold. Maybe the allure of BrainUp@ is powerful enough to give this strategy, medication for the whole population of symptom-free aging people, a push it doesn't deserve. Maybe the allure is so great that it chills assessment of the risk of prescribing any drug to that many people. Keep in mind that these potential patients are asymptomatic when they start the drug. This is not a question of balancing side effects of a drug versus the symptoms of a bad disease. This is balancing side effects of a drug you are taking for a disease you don't have.

And what are those risks? Polypharmacy, or regularly taking a wide array of prescription drugs, is a whopping problem for geriatric patients. Older people take many drugs, including ones that can be risky. In some studies the *mean* number of drugs prescribed to older patients is ten.[26] It is tough for anyone to take that many drugs exactly as prescribed, and even more so if you can't read small print or open bottles easily. Those drugs interact with one another and cause more problems, including falls, fractures, hospitalizations, and delirium. So one significant concern with the BrainUp@ strategy is that it's not a trivial matter to add yet another drug to the bucketfuls that older people already take. Good geriatricians and pharmacists spend a lot of time trying to whittle down prescriptions, and here comes BrainUp@ piling on.

BrainUp@ is also going to be expensive, not just for individual elders, but for the teeming aging population. A modest price would be $10,000 per year; $40,000 a year is not unlikely, multiplied by decades. Multiplied by the cohort of baby boomers, that's serious money: many billions. For those over sixty-five, that's money that comes out of Medicare, and therefore tax dollars. That's money we won't be able to use to rehab our aging housing stock so elders can keep living at home. We can't use it for physical therapy to optimize mobility or to promote exercise, healthy diets, and social engagement, all things that delay dementia. The people likely to take BrainUp@ will be old. They'll have other medical problems, like diabetes, cardiovascular disease, and cancer. They'll need lots of help. But we'll have spent a lot of money on the disease they don't have.

Let's look at one big clinical trial that treats those with preclinical Alzheimer's disease to try to slow or prevent dementia's onset. This is the BrainUp@ strategy in action. This clinical trial is A4, and its leadership features celebrated Alzheimer's experts, including Reisa Sperling and Jason Karlawish.[27] This trial will cost more than $100 million and take years and considerable manpower to complete. A4 will use PET scans to make sure everyone in the trial has excess amyloid. Participants will be evaluated to make sure they don't have dementia symptoms. The lack of symptoms but presence of excess amyloid means participants meet criteria for preclinical Alzheimer's. Some participants will get a placebo and others will get the active drug. At the start and at the end, all will get cognitive testing. Researchers will discover whether there is a difference in the number of people who develop worse cognitive function based on whether they got the drug or the placebo. The goal is to slow the onset of dementia.

Biogen has raised hopes with a similarly designed study using a different drug, aducanumab, due to be completed in 2019. The pilot study in March 2015 showed statistically significant decreases in amyloid and a slower rate of cognitive decline in those receiving the active drug. Aducanumab is not without side effects, including one with the mellifluous name of ARIA, for amyloid-related imaging abnormalities. ARIA refers to swelling of the brain, which got worse as the dose increased, and was more severe in those with the risk-increasing APOE e4. Still, this pilot study provided good news for Biogen, whose stock increased 40 percent in value over just a few months on the strength of early reports on this drug.[28] Subsequently, Biogen added five hundred more patients to the trial, suggesting concerns about the study and creating anxiety in market analysts.[29]

A lot is riding on the A4 trial. But there are reasons for concern. The drug being tested is solanezumab, or sola, the same one we already know doesn't help people with moderate or severe Alzheimer's. We also know that sola does not help the large group who look like they have Alzheimer's but don't have excess amyloid plaques. That's a lot of people who could use some help and won't get it from sola. The group that might have been helped by that $100 million study gets smaller and smaller.

In November 2016, Eli Lilly announced that sola had failed again. An extension of the fizzled trial of 2014 permitted sola to be studied just in research participants with amyloid proven by PET scan and mild impairment due to Alzheimer's. There was no clinically significant benefit for those receiving the active drug as opposed to the placebo. Lilly grimly noted in its press release that it "will not pursue regulatory submissions for solanezumab for the treatment of mild dementia due to Alzheimer's disease."[30] But neither sola nor A4 have been abandoned yet. A4 researchers, spying a nonsignificant blip toward improvement in an earlier trial, chose to *quadruple* the planned dose and extend the observation period for up to five years, hoping to fan that tiny spark of hope into a successful trial.[31] The results of the A4 trial are not yet ready, but so far, hundreds of millions of dollars have proved that sola does not help a lot of people with dementia. Could it delay symptoms in those who are symptom-free and only have amyloid plaques? This remains a theoretical possibility, but not one that inspires much confidence.

The tide has turned. It is hard today to wring funding out of NIH if your approach is all amyloid all the time. You need something more. Perhaps, you will say, this is science doing its job. A promising pathway was explored, and it just didn't work out. Now it's time to turn to other promising pathways. And while that's true, that description is too forgiving. Here's a quote from 2000 from Bill Thies, then a vice president of the Alzheimer's Association: "Either the beta-amyloid hypothesis is correct, in which case new therapies should come very quickly, or it isn't, in which case researchers at major laboratories will very quickly switch their efforts to more productive theories."[32] And let's compare that quote to one by Paul Aisen, director of the Alzheimer's Therapeutic Research Institute of the University of Southern California, commenting in 2016 on the latest failure of solanezumab. Aisen tells us, "This is not a refutation of the amyloid hypothesis . . . I think this is a confirmation of the amyloid hypothesis. I think it is the strongest confirmation to date."[33] Aisen is one of the foremost proponents of the amyloid hypothesis, and he shows no signs of backing down. With every failed trial there is a new explanation of why the drug didn't work but the hypothesis is still sound. Maybe the dose was too low or the intervention too late. Or maybe this isn't the right amyloid-lowering drug. Or maybe the trial showed a little bump in the right direction, but it just didn't reach statistical significance. Any of these things might be true in a particular trial, but they don't really get at the larger picture, which is that a lot of time and money have gone into explaining why the amyloid hypothesis has failed to benefit patients.

The truth is, amyloid is neither necessary nor sufficient for dementia. Solomon Fuller, who did work patiently and alone in his lab, knew this when he looked under his microscope a century ago. He found only weak correlations between the presence of plaques and dementia. Contemporary studies confirm that a large portion, 30 to 50 percent, of older people who die without dementia have significant amounts of amyloid in their brains.[34] Evidence like this has been available since Alzheimer's time, but researchers didn't always know what to do with it. Lorrie Moore captures something of this problem of not knowing what to make of what you see in her story "People Like That Are the Only People Here":[35]

> These imaging machines! They are like dogs, or metal detectors: they find everything, but don't know what they've found. That's where the surgeons come in. They're like the owners of the dogs. "Give me that," they say to the dog. "What the heck is that?"

This problem brings us close to the core of how science works. If you listen only to scientists discussing their hopes and wishes, we'd have cured a lot more things by now. We need trials and data to show the difference between something we hope will work and something that doesn't. You can't subject millions of people to the risk and expense of a drug that almost works. Advocates for the amyloid hypothesis raise reasonable questions, but after twenty-five years, it is time for different questions, including ones that look at other pathways, or even pathways that address amyloid without focusing on lowering it. But we have had trouble moving on. Why? Mostly because scientists and their funders are human. They build a career on a body of work. They stake their claim on proving their path is the right one.

Back in the 1930s, psychologist Gordon Allport described motives that acquired *functional autonomy*. He wrote of "rats trained to follow a long and difficult path, [who] will for a time persist in using this path, even though a short easy path to the goal is offered and even after the easier path has been learned."[36] What was once a means to an end becomes an end in itself. We are all like that rat at various points, and follow routes in our lives that have taken on functional autonomy. Zaven Khachaturian, the father of Alzheimer's research, argues that the amyloid hypothesis has attained functional autonomy.[37] It matters that Khachaturian raises these doubts. It signals deep reflection from a wise man with a long career. He is one of the last remaining of the generation of Alzheimer's researchers from the 1970s. He helped win early support for the amyloid hypothesis, and he is not denying that amyloid has a role in Alzheimer's. But we have been mesmerized. We need to look around and see what else is happening. We need to check out other pathways. None of this requires us to throw away all that has been learned, but we need to move on.

Scientists have trouble knowing what the heck to make of amyloid. Some people have disabling symptoms but only a modest amount of amyloid. Others have lots of amyloid and don't have symptoms. Some researchers try to minimize this discrepancy by claiming either that those amyloid-heavy people would get dementia if we just waited or that they already have subtle deficits we are missing. Alas for that argument, there are centenarians with excess amyloid and fine cognition. In fact, if I can make it to a hundred with only minimal problems, sign me up.

The most widely accepted explanation for the disjunction between amyloid and symptoms is offered by Yaakov Stern, director of Neuro-cognitive Science at Columbia. Stern is a tall, thin, graying professor with large glasses and a jolly demeanor. He uses the concept of *cognitive reserve* to explain why some individuals tolerate heavy brain pathology, including amyloid plaques, while preserving good cognitive function.[38] An individual with high cognitive reserve draws upon multiple brain networks and other compensatory mechanisms to maintain function despite growing levels of brain injury. Stern's evidence shows that cognitive reserve differs between haves and have-nots. As in other domains of health, privilege begets privilege; them what has gits. If you have more education and a job that uses it, you tolerate a higher level of brain pathology before you develop symptoms. There is a downside to this privilege. When those with high cognitive reserve do develop symptoms of dementia, they go downhill faster than those with less reserve. It seems that those compensatory mechanisms cover up real damage. Once compensation is exhausted, a tipping point is reached and decline comes quickly. Getting an education, exercising, and staying intellectually and socially engaged all contribute to cognitive reserve. They don't prevent dementia, but may slow down the appearance of its symptoms. I asked Dr. Stern what he does to maintain his own cognitive reserve, and he admitted that finding time to exercise is a problem, given his busy work schedule. At least he tries to walk up the stairs to his office every day. I asked, "Aren't you on the eighteenth floor?" "It's really nineteen, but still, I should do more." His example may not be easy to follow, but his point is well taken. You can't change your genes, but you can work on cognitive reserve, and should get busy about it.

Dementia specialists realize the unfairness of the link between better health, better education, and jobs. Kristine Yaffe is vice chair of Research in Psychiatry at UCSF and a world-renowned dementia researcher. She has an easy smile and laid-back California style that belie a fearsome work ethic; she completed residencies in both psychiatry and neurology to make sure she had the best possible training. Yaffe points out the discomfort that researchers experience in studying disparities in cognitive health outcomes tied to class. "There seem to be quite striking differences in outcomes in diverse populations. It doesn't seem to be the rate of cognitive change so much as it is where people are starting, and where people are starting influences where they end up. Nobody wants to tackle these differences."[39] This is the impact of the social determinants of health. This is perhaps the biggest of all ethical problems in medicine. It cannot be solved by a strategy focused on medication alone, but requires changing the access to factors that promote health in all areas of a patient's life.

What should people do today about dementia? Can testing help? That contentious issue boiled over in a squabble about the appropriate use of special PET scans that detect amyloid. Advocates, including the Alzheimer's Association and Eli Lilly, which makes the radioactive molecule used in the tests, urged Medicare to cover the cost of these scans so people could find out their amyloid status. A person who knew she was likely to develop Alzheimer's might want to get her papers in order, think about long-term care insurance, and examine her living situation with an eye to future disability. But the presence of amyloid does not tell us when or even if a person will develop dementia. This crucial distinction was lost in most of the reporting around the coverage decision; in fact, reporters consistently referred to the scan as an "Alzheimer's test," though it does not measure whether a person has dementia. The federal government declined to cover the cost of these scans unless the person agreed to enroll in a research protocol. This was the right decision.[40]

Some experts disagreed, and they banded together to form the IDEAS study, supported by the Alzheimer's Association.[41] Preliminary results were reported in a triumphal tone; roughly two-thirds of patients received changes in prescribed dementia or other medications and/or counseling after their PET scans. For the researchers, this proved the clear benefit of PET scans. Although I respect the significant clinical experience and wisdom of those involved in the trial, I'm not a believer. A PET scan reveals whether you have excess amyloid. If you have too much, you are at higher risk of dementia, but we don't know when or if you'll get it. If you don't have too much amyloid, you may *still* get dementia. The PET scan says nothing about your function, including whether you are developing symptoms of dementia or its precursor, minimal cognitive impairment. Neuropsychological testing could tell you that, but being able to avoid that is one of the supposed advantages of having a PET scan. If you are impaired, the test can't tell which medicines are better for you or when your symptoms will progress. I am puzzled by what information it could provide that helps doctors change treatment. I would prefer a thorough assessment of my function, counseling that addresses those findings, and medicines that might help address my symptoms, and the PET scan sheds no light on any of that.

A PET scan offers a lot of "scienciness," a concept I've adapted from Stephen Colbert's concept of "truthiness," defined as something that feels true but is not. If you get a picture of the amyloid in your brain, you feel you have scientific information. But you really just have a "sciencey" picture that doesn't tell you more, or perhaps as much, as your family history. If PET scans can be marketed as "Alzheimer's tests," worried people will waste their money on them, without gaining much real information about their risk of dementia, or putting that money to better use in buying fruits and vegetables or making sure their home will accommodate them if dementia develops.

But why not let people get the scan if they can pay for it? Because there are some real liabilities to this action. Alzheimer's is a devastating disease, greatly stigmatized. Insurance companies can prevent a person with demonstrated amyloid buildup or "preclinical Alzheimer's disease" from buying long-term care insurance or life insurance, since preexisting conditions are not protected for those types of insurance. And what would an employer do who learned an employee had "preclinical Alzheimer's disease"? Progress in preventing other diseases has followed from encouraging clinicians and patients to watch out for prediabetes and precancerous growths. There is nothing inherently wrong in tracking signs that a disease may be brewing. The warning sign may not always produce the disease; not every scary skin lesion turns into melanoma. But the stigma and fear associated with Alzheimer's dementia are especially onerous. Reisa Sperling has been one of the major proponents of creating the preclinical category, yet she comments, "I understand the ethical concerns about labeling someone when we don't have the enlightenment in the world that Alzheimer's disease does not necessarily mean someone curled up in a ball in a nursing home."[42] Studying those in the preclinical category to see if we can prevent severe disease and change that image is a key goal for Dr. Sperling. For now, knowing your amyloid status won't predict whether you'll develop dementia, but it can show that you have an elevated risk. As many as 40 percent of people develop dementia by the age of eighty-five. I have a family history of the disease, so I assume I'll be in that group. A PET scan won't give me better data than that.

Of all the things I've read about dementia, the Nun Study sticks with me as much as anything. It's so simple. And it brilliantly illustrates what we don't know about dementia. The Nun Study (that's actually its name) looked at 678 Catholic sisters, aged 75 to 107.[43] The researchers combed through convent archives, reviewing essays the sisters had written in their youth. The study also included annual physical and cognitive exams for as long as the sisters lived. And when they died, the good sisters donated their brains to science so that others might benefit from their generosity. We have.

Besides some very appealing portraits of older women, the study offers compelling information about aging. Underscoring the importance of a good start, those sisters who scored high on measures of cognitive strength in youth continued to do so in old age. But the central finding is that people display an incredible range of symptoms, imperfectly correlated to their plaques and tangles. Some nuns have none (sorry), while others have a lot, even with the same location, type, and amount of pathology. Sister Bernadette is typical; she died at eighty-five with lots of plaques and tangles, but no dementia symptoms. This is the central mystery of dementia. Amyloid and tau are doing something, but the way they affect people changes radically from person to person. If you have strokes, those plaques and tangles are more likely to lead to symptoms. If you have more education or a protective APOE e2 gene, then you can tolerate more damage.[44] It may not be that we need to lower amyloid, but that we need to figure out how to live better with it. Some of us can do that. The rest of us would be very happy to learn their secret.

There is an additional problem in the relationship of amyloid to Alzheimer's. We know there are people who have symptoms that look like Alzheimer's but who don't have excess amyloid. Likewise, there are people who have lots of amyloid but don't have symptoms. Today, if a person has excess amyloid and dementia, it is assumed that amyloid is the cause. But logically, that cannot always be true. If you can have dementia without amyloid and amyloid without dementia, then at least some people with both amyloid and dementia have a dementia that is not related to amyloid. The way Alzheimer's is defined, the way it insists on amyloid, and the way our research protocols are configured, we cannot see those people today. We have erased a category of people with dementia from our definitions and our studies; in fact, we have designed our categories to ignore their existence. A lot of research will be necessary to clarify the puzzling relationships between amyloid and dementia before it becomes worthwhile for you to invest in a scan.

I asked Yaakov Stern, for whom dementia runs in the family, whether he thought PET scans and other tests, including APOE e4, were useful today for helping patients make decisions about dementia. He replied: "For myself, I'm not interested. I could get any study done, working here [at Columbia]—I could probably get it done and not have to pay for it. This is an incredible research center and every test is done here by one of my colleagues—genetic studies, PET, MRI. I don't want any of the tests. I don't know what any of them means. They don't tell me what to do. They're not helpful to me as an individual in any way."[45]

I agree with Dr. Stern. Given my family's history, I know I am at risk and that a healthy lifestyle may decrease that risk. There is no other step I can take, and no information can alter that knowledge. And too much information is not always helpful. If I chose to get APOE e4 testing, I might learn I have one copy of the gene, confirming the risk I already know. Or I might learn I have two copies. I'd find that depressing, and it might actually undermine my efforts to stay healthy. If I didn't have APOE e4, wouldn't that be cause for celebration? Nope. The *majority* of people with Alzheimer's dementia don't have the APOE e4 gene. A clean bill of health could create a falsely rosy view. My family history remains the best information available.

The setbacks for the amyloid hypothesis have generated a resurgence for Tauists, and not without a certain crowing on their part.[46] In fact, the amount and location of tau in the brain correlate much better with dementia symptoms than amyloid does. And while only about a third of older people accumulate amyloid, almost everyone over seventy has abnormal tau in their brain. As Sperling notes, "Everyone has a little tau, but they don't get demented unless the tau spreads, and the tau doesn't spread unless there is amyloid."[47] Which is the chicken and which is the egg? There is something essential yet to be worked out.

There are some intriguing clues as to what that something might be. Yale researchers in 2017 restored synapses and improved memory in mice, not by lowering amyloid in the brain, but by preventing binding between amyloid and a specific receptor, thus preventing the transmission of harmful information into the neuron.[48] So maybe we don't need to lower amyloid so much as keep it from harming neurons. But here is a major caveat: An entire book could be filled with such tantalizing clues. This study is not yet close to being tested in humans; it has not even gotten as far as the 99.6 percent failure rate. As Dr. Joe Verghese commented about a different mouse study, "We have cured Mouseheimer's over and over. We have trouble translating the work to humans."[49]

The best way to summarize the state of research regarding amyloid, tau, and dementia today is one of creative confusion, awaiting a significant breakthrough. The amyloid hypothesis isn't dead exactly, but it is old and frail. It is also evolving. Perhaps it is only some types of amyloid that do the dirty work, or maybe injuries to the aging brain make it tougher to get rid of amyloid. Maybe genetic risk factors bend some of us toward vulnerability in the presence of amyloid. I asked Kristine Yaffe how she conceptualized the different factors that add up to dementia in older people. She said:

> I think first of all it depends on age. I do think things change quite a bit as one gets older, in terms of mixed pathologies and maybe different mechanisms. Most likely it's a combination of things, multiple things. One enters old age with a backdrop of some hits, and those vary depending on the person's life and genetics and cognitive reserve. Has the person had a traumatic brain injury? Does the person have APOE e4? Does the person have high or low cognitive reserve? Or a chronic psychiatric disorder? Major cardiovascular risk factors? Diabetes? Those would be my biggies . . . Those are things you have had, and you are now seventy years old. Up until now that history hasn't manifested itself much as far as your brain. But now you take that history and your age and you meet what has been happening on a parallel path with the accumulation of protein in the brain, of tau and beta-amyloid. It's a complex mixture of all these things. The amount of tau and beta-amyloid you have by the time you were seventy is based a lot on your genetics, but also on some of these other hits. They interact with one another. People who get Alzheimer's in their forties and fifties are people who have autosomal dominant genes and have been just snowed with amyloid for the last two decades, and now they have Alzheimer's. But for the rest of us,

it starts later. It interacts with all the other comorbidities and less dominant genetics, and the traumatic brain injuries and mild strokes and lifelong depression. It all comes to the fore then. There are certain things that may interact to promote more protein accumulation or help the person withstand it— that's where cognitive reserve comes in. And then if one makes it to the eighties and nineties, then you may have a different pathology, which is even more of a mixed bag. You start to see a lot more of the vascular accumulation and less of a role for amyloid.[50]

Yaffe's statement, which she rattled off extemporaneously during our interview, is the best summary I've heard of how a brilliant scientist working now thinks about how we develop dementia in old age. It's not a single thing. It's not one gene. It's a life's worth of lottery tickets, some winners and some losers, whose numbers come up after decades. No single pill will fix it.

Dementia is not one disease. Alzheimer's is not even one disease, but a clinical syndrome—a batch of symptoms—caused by different processes in different people. People with one form of dementia have different brain changes from those with another. Many people have multiple types of brain changes contributing to dementia. Indeed, a common form of dementia shows both changes in blood vessels *and* the plaques and tangles of Alzheimer's.

People with dementia used to be part of a massive forest of patients with undesirable symptoms; their needs were barely distinguished. Now dementia is its own forest. But even so, we need to look within to identify the different types if we are to really make gains against it. And there are scientists who are doing this; they are picking apart the individual types of dementia the way a forester might walk through a wood and say, "Here is a shagbark hickory, that's a sassafras, and here is an ancient apple tree." Some interventions may help with any type of dementia, but others will affect only one and not another.

Solving the puzzle of dementia will take a village. No lonely hero will lift her head and holler, "Eureka!" Success will come incrementally, not like a thunderclap. If a clinical trial succeeds, it will bring some help to some people. It will be a start upon which researchers can build. Researchers are still trying to decrease the amount of amyloid in the brain, but there is now both excitement and funding for different approaches. That's a good thing even if an amyloid-lowering drug finally works. (I am not holding my breath, but hey, I don't know everything.) Different approaches—either other drugs or a well-tested exercise and diet program, or something completely different—could bolster a drug that works a bit, and somewhat bigger groups may benefit or bigger gains emerge. This model—the additive use of multiple interventions—is the one that has delivered the most medical successes in the last several decades. It is what has helped treat AIDS and made it into a chronic disease instead of a death sentence. It is how we approach many cancers and other serious illnesses. And as Reisa Sperling points out, a study like A4 doesn't have to cure dementia, "it just has to bend the curve. If you can just keep people asymptomatic for five more years, they will die out ballroom dancing rather than in a nursing home."[51]

I don't want to leave this topic without reporting some good news. There has been progress in slowing down dementia—it just hasn't come from a drug. The *percentage* of older people developing dementia is decreasing.[52] (Confusingly, the actual number of people newly diagnosed with dementia is still increasing, because so many more of us live into old age.) As Yaffe commented, "This is one of the few positive things we've heard, and the public health implications are enormous. It's not about Big Pharma developing a very expensive drug or getting a very sensitive CT scan. It's about public health issues, like improving public education, treating cardiovascular disease." This is great news and helps underscore the reasons to exercise, eat healthfully, and engage socially and intellectually. All those things help build cognitive reserve and protect brain function.

We need to question the stereotypic image of an octogenarian sitting quietly on the porch in a rocking chair. That might be the right choice for some, but we should update our expectations to include seniors who embark on new and thrilling projects. I met a bubbly retired hairdresser in her eighties who had recently taken up singing. She had never sung in public, but decided to give it a try. She was accepted into a class for professional singers. Perhaps they thought she was kind of a joke, with her diminutive height and smoky voice. But she took the work extremely seriously. She got better. She sang in public. She caught on. When I met her, she had just completed a successful solo cabaret performance at a posh Manhattan jazz club. She was bursting with pride about her burgeoning venture—she didn't expect to get rich, but she was having so much fun, making other people happy while singing jazz classics. She beamed when she described her renewed lease on life. An encore career as a singer wouldn't be the right choice for me. (Can you believe my husband has asked me not to sing in the shower? So hurtful.) But many older people enjoy learning and exploring, and they reap benefits when they do. You can't change your genes and you may not ultimately prevent dementia, but you might have more joy today and for more days and slow down dementia's onset by years.

Dementia creates a lot of anxiety, as do thoughts of aging in general. It doesn't have to be that way. Take a walk. Spend time with those you love. Sing. Eat fruits. Pick up a new skill or hobby. There is no guarantee these things will slow dementia's onset, but they are as good a bet as any. No matter what, they may increase your store of happiness along the way.

Chapter 9

Money, Money, Money

In the film *The Martian*, Matt Damon plays a plucky astronaut who gets stuck on Mars with dwindling food supplies and no hope of rescue for years. Bummer. What does he do? He never despairs. He sciences his way out. He figures out how to grow potatoes fertilized by his own shit. He survives long enough for friends to fly through space to his rescue. A happy ending ensues—yeah, plucky astronaut! But let's look at how our hero uses science to survive. He doesn't sit and wait for the expensive shiny machine to swoop in and rescue him— that way lies certain death. He goes old school, combining low-tech methods and creativity to bridge the gap between what he needs today and what he's hoping the future will bring. He uses his noggin, he uses his hands; technology is his servant, not his master.

We are trying to science our way out of the problem of dementia. We invest billions in finding magic pills so we can avoid the expense of caring for those who have it. If and when we get real treatments or prevention, that will be great. But a pill is not going to rescue the baby boomers. Between those already ill and those whose brains are developing pathological changes, we will have increasing numbers of people with dementia for twenty years or more—maybe much more. We better start planting potatoes. We'll have to apply a better portion of our research funding, our care dollars, and our best thinking to the problem of providing care.

Our national policy for the last thirty years could be summed up accordingly: It's smart to spend money on drug research so we can save money on care. The standard argument for funding research is that we must win this battle or we'll face unbearable expenses caring for the millions who will develop dementia as our population ages. We are already there. We can't dodge that bullet.

Here is a more realistic plan. First, stop pinning your hopes on a magic pill. Keep in mind that 99.6 percent failure rate for new dementia drugs. No new medications have emerged for fifteen years, and the ones we have are palliative at best. Second, successful treatment will require a multifaceted intervention, to address the multiple pathways to disease. That's how we've made progress in AIDS and cancer. We'll need not one but several wins—and we've had none at all. Third, those drugs are not free. Our success in treating cancer more than doubled the cost of cancer care in recent decades. It's great we have better cancer care, but that means we now spend a lot more on those treatments. They don't save money; they *cost* money. If we one day create a batch of drugs that diminish dementia's symptoms, that will also be great, but they won't save us money. (They will likely make somebody very rich.)

Most important, even if we find drugs that work, we'll still need to care for people with dementia for many years. Here's why: The brain pathology that causes dementia forms over decades. It takes roughly ten years to get a new drug to the market. In that time, millions more will develop dementia. And if drugs successfully slow disease progression, we may need to care for *more* people with dementia, since survival will increase. We will have even more older people living longer, with disability, and needing care and support.

Supporters of drug research will object to my comments, arguing that we need more, not fewer pharmaceutical studies. They're not entirely wrong—as a physician, I support continued research for dementia, including in pharmacology. We've seen failure after failure in these drug trials, yes, but that is not what worries me. We already know there won't be a dementia cure in time for millions of baby boomers. I'm worried about our failure to create a realistic national policy to provide and pay for dementia care. If we focused more on the reality of care and less on the fantasy of eradication, we might at last deal with these pressing issues.

A plan for care must be empathic, affordable, and flexible. Science is not just about shiny machines; it is about using evidence to fix important problems. How can we devise a viable strategy to pay for long-term care? How do we preserve dignity? How do we balance freedom and safety? What is a good death for someone with dementia? How can we use technology and funds wisely, combining care with comfort, choice, and dignity?

On a lovely May morning, Dr. Mirnova Ceide and I arrive at an apartment building to meet Mrs. B, an older woman with dementia. There are four steps to get to the main door of the building and four steps up from the lobby to her first-floor apartment. For Mrs. B and her family, these eight steps loom large, since she can no longer walk. Getting her in or out of the apartment requires multiple helpers, and is risky and painful for her. A lot of the housing stock in New York City—indeed, in America—is old and tough to navigate for those with disabilities. Waiting lists for accessible housing are years long.

For a frail elder like Mrs. B, the waiting list is longer than her predicted life-span. She will live out her days here if she can. Since she cannot easily come and go, home visits are a lifeline. Dr. Ceide is a specialist in geriatric psychiatry and an assistant professor at Einstein and Montefiore, where I work. Part of her job is visiting these members of the community at their homes.

Outside it is sunny; inside, the light is crepuscular. The Virgin Mary presides from a shelf. Religious images adorn every wall. Mrs. B is so tiny she disappears beneath the blankets on the hospital bed in the living room. She lives here with her partner of many years. An aide visits for eight hours, five days a week. Mr. and Mrs. B speak Spanish, though Mr. B and the aide speak limited English as well. Mrs. B also has severe hearing loss. Dr. Ceide emanates warmth and generates trust. She is a great communicator, but we face a communication difficulty, as Dr. Ceide speaks little Spanish. Decades ago, I spoke Spanish in a childlike yet fluent fashion, but now my skills are rusty. We have access to translators over the phone; but cell phone access in the community is spotty, and for a person who is hard of hearing and demented, a three-way phone conversation is bewildering—technology doesn't solve all communication challenges. Quixotically, I plunge into the breach with my faulty Spanish.

My attempt to administer a mental status exam resembles an especially insensitive comedy sketch. I yell instructions in halting Spanish, and Mrs. B looks puzzled. The aide then leans down next to her ear and yells the instructions in louder and better Spanish. Mrs. B does her best to follow along, repeating three words or naming the objects in front of her. The devoted aide automatically adapts the tasks to make them easier. For example, I say in bad Spanish, "Raise your right hand, touch your nose, open your mouth," to see if Mrs. B can recall complex instructions. The aide lovingly leans down and yells, "Raise your right hand, my darling," which Mrs. B does. Then the aide says, "Very good, my angel! Touch your nose. Good! You are doing so well, my love!", and then "Open your mouth, my dear heart." It was a fine demonstration of how to provide loving care to a vulnerable patient, but not a valid medical test. The exam shows Mrs. B can focus for brief periods and that her memory is badly impaired; it is hard to say more than that.

We learn that Mrs. B needs total care. She wears a diaper. She can no longer walk. The aide gets her out of bed to sit up in a chair as much as possible. This family's biggest trouble is that for months now, Mrs. B has been up a lot at night, crying and calling for Mr. B to help her. She can neither see nor hear well, and nights are scary. She is frightened of being alone, frightened that Mr. B has gone, and frightened of what may happen to her. She is less frightened during the day. His presence comforts her; hers also comforts him. Mr. B clearly loves Mrs. B, but he is eighty-two and exhausted from running into the living room multiple times every night. They have been together fifty-five years. He says to her quietly, not unkindly, "Should I go?" and Mrs. B is instantly tearful, revealing a tiny glimpse of the nightly drama of her cries and laments. Of course, the aide is there during the day, but this infirm and aging couple desperately need someone to help them at night.

Dr. Ceide reviews all the medicines on the side table and says she will try to get them help at night. Mrs. B has always been religious, and Dr. Ceide thinks she may be able to find a local priest who does home visits, to diminish their isolation. Mr. and Mrs. B and the aide all give us warm handshakes as we leave, and ask that God watch over us.

One of the most frequent reasons a family can no longer keep a person with dementia at home is that he or she has disturbed sleep patterns, and the family, often an equally elderly partner, grow exhausted from tending to nighttime crises. The B family is right on the edge of this precipice. Mrs. B would like to stay home as she ages, rather than go to a nursing facility. This is true of many people, rich or poor, whether their home is a magnificent estate or a walk-up apartment. Mr. B agrees that this home, where they have lived so long, is the right place for her. Still, the sleepless nights are wearing him out fast. Mrs. B is eligible for Medicaid, which provides her daytime aide. These aides are not easy to get, and many people need more help at home than Medicaid will pay for. This is true even in New York, which has more generous coverage than most states. Maybe Mrs. B and her family won't get additional help, and she will end up in a facility. They don't want that. New York State doesn't want that, either, because the cost of care in a nursing home is $85,000 a year and up. But round-the-clock care at home costs even more. Medicaid does not pay for that.

Geriatrician Amy Ehrlich is a widely admired clinician and medical director of Montefiore Home Care, a certified home health agency. She sees a lot of families like the Bs, struggling to help keep a relative at home. I asked her what ethical dilemmas these families faced. She said, "Let's call a spade a spade. It's got nothing to do with ethics. It's got to do with economics . . . It's much cheaper to have someone in a medical institution than someone at home" once they need twenty-four-hour care.[1] Every day Dr. Ehrlich faces questions about what it means to support elders at home once they need this level of care. She and I are old friends; we have had heated and intense discussions since we were heated and intense Harvard freshmen, our 1970s tresses like Amazon jungle vines. I pushed back, arguing that fiscal policies *are* ethical choices about how we as a community and a nation choose to spend money. Ethics, money, safety, and quality of life are woven together.

Dr. Ehrlich notes that it's not only Medicaid patients who must do without services they need to safely live at home. One of her patients had just barely too much money to qualify for Medicaid; she was almost blind and cognitively impaired. She proudly told Dr. Ehrlich that her rabbi allowed her to start lighting candles early on the Sabbath. "Why was that?" Dr. Ehrlich inquired. Because the woman's failed vision meant she really didn't know if she was lighting a candle or something else, maybe the curtains—and she liked to take her time. Horrified, Dr. Ehrlich phoned the rabbi to point out the very real dangers for this patient and her neighbors. Could he tell her patient it was against Jewish law for her to light candles? Could she find a helper or use battery-operated fake candles? Amy is a master at cobbling together resources to keep her patients at home without jeopardizing their safety (or their neighbors').

New York State's policy is to reduce the number of people in nursing homes. They are tightening requirements for nursing home placement, reducing reimbursement, and nudging the industry toward fewer available beds. The B family's problem is typical for dementia care. Many people say they would like to stay at home and age in place. The state and taxpayers like to support freedom of choice, and also like the sound of avoiding expensive nursing homes. But these people need services, and those cost money. When ought we to say that for this person, no matter his or her preferences, it is time for institutional care? And what determines that decision—is it when needs are so great we simply can't ensure safety? Or when we just don't like the price of doing so? The B family faces practical questions of what help Medicaid will provide. Dr. Ehrlich raises crucial questions for the rest of us. How much cost is too much to help someone stay home? And what kinds of cost matter in our accounting: Do we count the cost of splitting up Mr. and Mrs. B, of forcing her away from her home and family? How much benefit justifies how much expense?

Certainly paying for the care of disabled people is not a new problem. In the nineteenth century, state officials built an armada of mental hospitals on the premise that cure would follow and costs would go down. That didn't work. After World War II, government placed frail elders in nursing homes rather than mental hospitals, hoping they could get by with less expensive "custodial" care. That didn't work either. Many now advocate for dementia's cure because care is just too expensive. So far we have no cure, and there is none in sight. Furthermore, we have no reasonable expectation that the need for and cost of care will go down. Providing good care for those with chronic needs is expensive, and it's going to stay that way. It is ethically possible, even advisable, to look at ways to spend money prudently without sacrificing quality and dignity. But to claim you've found a way to get out of paying such costs, either through cure or by shifting the burden elsewhere, just doesn't work. So what would be an effective way to provide and pay for care for elders with dementia?

Appealing solutions change over time. Policies that pushed frail elders with disabilities into nursing facilities had many problems, including the fact that institutions restrict a person's liberty. Freedom for the disabled didn't have much weight as a policy concept some decades ago, but various civil rights movements—for minorities, women, patients, the mentally ill, and the disabled—all coalesced into a wider recognition of universal rights. National policy received a significant push in the direction of liberty with the 1999 U.S. Supreme Court Olmstead decision, which found that disabled persons had a right to have their needs met in the least restrictive setting possible. No longer would it be acceptable to admit someone to an institution whose needs could be met in the community.[2] This decision forced a reexamination of many policies and provided huge support to community-based agencies that could help make life with disability a reality outside an institution. *Olmstead* opened a new era in which the preferences and values of disabled persons mattered.

This focus on autonomy was a big step forward ethically. But implementing those preferences raises equally complex issues. What are the costs, financial and personal, of supporting someone with disabilities at home, rather than in an institution? Does the state have a right to say that costs above a certain amount or under certain circumstances are too great to pay? And are there limits to the costs that family members should pay, both monetary and more broadly conceived? For Mr. and Mrs. B, should Medicaid pay for more help at home, even if those costs exceed that of nursing home care? Or maybe we need more access to different options, maybe some housing in which Mr. and Mrs. B could stay together, but in which health professionals would provide better backup? All across the country, families and providers face questions with serious ethical challenges. What is desirable from whose perspective? What is feasible? What is the best balance— for this specific family and for the whole population—of freedom, safety, and fiscal responsibility?

Deinstitutionalization of patients with mental illness produced devastating consequences because adequate community support networks never materialized. Current efforts to keep people with dementia out of the nursing home raise worrisome comparisons. Will states supply the necessary services so these elders can live safely at home? Today's health policy advocates are working hard to put the right supports in place and avoid history's repeating itself. But policy wonks don't control funds. In a time of small government, it is hard to set up new safety net programs. Many already exist or are in development, but the extent to which they work and for whom is still under study. So far, the evidence is mixed about the extent of potential savings when those with dementia dwell in the community with the support to do that safely.

The cost of caring for those with dementia is staggering. The best estimate, from a 2010 study led by Michael Hurd for the Rand Corporation, concluded that it was roughly $200 billion yearly, making it one of our most expensive diseases.[3] This sum will only increase in the coming years. We are growing older as a society. More of us are demented. Medical research will not eradicate that truth any time soon, not before many more of us develop dementia. Indeed, successful treatment may slow its progress, meaning more people will remain in the mild to moderate phase for longer, and thus require support for longer, and there will be more of them. We are not ready to care for them.

A substantial percentage of Medicaid costs are for elders in nursing homes. There is a big push politically to decrease those costs, in part by eliminating long-term beds. Some facilities are closing altogether, and some are converting their beds from long-term care to the more lucrative short-term rehabilitation beds covered by Medicare. The goal is to encourage elders, including those with dementia, to age at home. But providing meaningful support outside of institutions requires real funding for community services. For people like Mrs. B, that support costs more than a nursing home. And autonomy looks less appealing to bean counters once it costs more than an institution. But here is where our policies are at cross-purposes. We don't like the expense of nursing homes, so we are cutting back beds. But we like even less the greater expense of full support at home for frail, demented elders. We are decreasing nursing home beds and setting limits on services at home, and the population of frail, demented elders continues to grow. We are setting up a riptide for America's Mrs. Bs.

Many Americans assume that long-term care for the elderly in a nursing home or by attendants at home is covered by Medicare, but Medicare does not cover the cost of long-term care. Medicare covers *short-term* rehabilitation in a nursing home, as well as temporary assistance at home, but not long-term services. Instead, Medicaid pays more than 60 percent of long-term care costs.[4] But that's odd, since Medicaid covers only those with low incomes. Surely, by definition, most Americans must be middle class and not eligible for that kind of support. The sad truth is that our failure to develop a coherent national plan to pay for long-term care drives huge numbers of older Americans into poverty. Indeed, one might describe our national policy as a perversion of the Shakespearean adage: Some are born poor, some become poor, and some have poverty thrust upon them. We encourage elders to become poor, and if that doesn't work, we thrust poverty upon them.

Consider the case of Rita Sherman, as described by journalist Ron Lieber.[5] Ms. Sherman did everything right. She saved carefully, retiring with more than $600,000, and bought a long-term care policy that would cover up to three years of care. By the time she died at ninety-four, after more than five years of living in a nursing home, it was all gone. For her final years, she was forced to rely on Medicaid. She planned well, lived within her means, and took every step recommended to provide for her old age. It was not enough. And Mrs. Sherman is not the only one. We live much longer with disability than any prior generation. When the retirement age was set at sixty-five, people lived until seventy. Now many of us live until ninety or beyond. *Aesop's Fables* tell us of the grasshopper who partied hard all summer and the ant who stocked up against the coming winter. The grasshopper must beg when cold weather comes, while the ant feels morally superior and has plenty. In the system we have today, even ants go begging. The costs of care are much higher, for longer, than the most cautious ant could save for.

Many question whether families could do more to help demented elders. A look at the data is sobering. Families already provide an extraordinary amount of uncompensated care for disabled older family members. Of the roughly $200 billion of dementia's annual cost, Medicare pays only $11 billion. Care contributed by unpaid family members is by far the single greatest source.[6] Of the more than 2 million caregivers who watch over dying elders in the United States yearly, nine out of ten are unpaid.[7]

Couldn't elders save more to pay for their own care? Our current policies, with rare exceptions, actively discourage saving for long-term care. Instead, elder law specialists across the country advise their clients to "spend down"—that is to say, burn through savings until they are impoverished and qualify for Medicaid. Medicaid policies were formerly so draconian that they sometimes forced into homelessness the spouses of those who needed long-term care. Now many states permit couples to sequester their primary residence, up to a certain point, from those assets that count in the assessment of eligibility for Medicaid. And some innovations permit elders to shelter additional assets, while still meeting eligibility for Medicaid long-term care above a certain cost.[8]

Forcing middle-class people into poverty and then relying on programs for the poor to cover long-term care costs is unsustainable. As more and more of us become older and develop dementia, we won't all fit in the leaky lifeboat of Medicaid. Already, Medicaid is the single largest item in New York State's budget, accounting for nearly a third of costs, more than either education or transportation.[9] Those who wish to cut Medicaid often portray recipients as able-bodied adults who choose not to work. In truth, a huge part of the Medicaid budget is for elders with dementia in nursing homes. They cannot get out of bed; they are incontinent; they can't feed themselves. Often they have outlived all family members. We'll face even greater need going forward. We have a growing population of those who will need long-term care, and we are not prepared to care for them.

Americans who are neither very poor nor very rich are increasingly aware of the financial risks they face. They eagerly seek solutions. Very few of us have retirement funds sufficient to pay for five years of nursing home care, after we've lived in retirement for decades, but a minority of us may require just that. So why not get insurance in case expenses spiral out of control? Long-term care insurance holds intuitive appeal, but is not a viable option for many today. Fifteen years ago, more than a hundred companies sold long-term care insurance, which was a relatively new product and thought to have a bright future. The ideal purchaser, from the company's point of view, was a healthy adult in his fifties, not ready to retire but old enough to begin planning. This not-yet-old adult might be able to lock in a low annual fee for long-term care insurance, given the small likelihood he would need to make a claim against the policy that year. Insurance is a one-year product; you spend money for coverage this year, and if you don't make a claim, that money is gone forever. You buy insurance again next year, and so forth and so forth until you need long-term care and claim your benefits. A person at fifty is unlikely to require long-term care that year, so few will buy unless there is some sweetener. Both buyer and seller realize that in twenty years, when the buyer is in his seventies, the probability of needing the policy will be far greater. Factors that encourage early purchase include low cost and the ability to lock in a low price for the future by buying when healthy.

Insurance companies took a beating. For several reasons, they were seriously off in their calculations of how much they'd need to earn in premiums to cover claims. Elder care costs increased rapidly. Interest rates went to historic lows, so companies saw little profit from the funds they held. Mortality from stroke, heart disease, and cancer has decreased, but we survive those conditions with chronic disabilities and need assistance with eating, eliminating, and moving around. As claims skyrocketed, sellers of long-term care insurance sustained epic losses; one major seller of long-term care insurance saw the value of its stock fall by 50 percent in a year.[10] Insurance companies petitioned regulators for increases in premiums. For some elderly consumers, the cost of long-term care insurance—totally separate from medical insurance—approaches $7,000 yearly.[11] The likelihood that annual costs will stay low even for someone who bought early is dwindling.

The insurance companies don't want your business. They are getting out of long-term care in droves. The annual cost of policies has increased, and the ability to buy one has decreased. Any information on preexisting medical conditions can and will be used against you. (The Affordable Care Act protects consumers with preexisting conditions when buying *health* insurance, but that protection does not apply to long-term care or life insurance.) There has been a lot of debate about why so few seniors buy long-term care insurance.[12] It's hardly a mystery. The policies are expensive, they cover too little, and too many people are excluded. Gender inequities rear their ugly head, too. Men are less likely to need paid long-term care, as they are more likely to have a spouse who provides unpaid care. This means that policies for men are less expensive and easier to get. Women pose a greater risk for needing long-term care, since they live longer, often outlive a spouse, and are less likely to have that spouse provide care. The payback for women's commitment to care is that policies are more expensive and harder to get. A small percentage of people currently hold long-term care policies; their numbers will not grow unless and until something major changes. For now, the market for private long-term care insurance is in trouble.

Could the federal government solve this problem? Not easily, though this remains the most likely source of a solution. The Affordable Care Act (ACA) tried to tackle it. The late senator Ted Kennedy sponsored a provision in the ACA to help pay for long-term care through the Community Living Assistance Services and Supports Act (CLASS Act), which proposed voluntary contributions from consumers and supplements from the government.[13] The Congressional Budget Office estimated its costs far higher than the sponsors had. That bad news put a stake through its heart, and the CLASS Act died shortly after its main defender, Senator Kennedy. Frankly, even those who advocated for long-term care had doubts about the CLASS Act. Most experts do not believe that voluntary contributions could ever cover the likely costs. What would work instead is a plan that includes a wide range of people, young and old, and is mandatory. The chances of creating this new safety net are currently between zero and invisibly small. We are creating an insoluble problem for the generation who must care for today's baby boomers.

There is an army of health policy mavens working on these issues, trying to control costs and provide care. I met many of them when I was lucky enough to spend a year as a Health and Aging Policy Fellow.[14] This program pairs experts in aging with government agencies and other groups; the government gets free expertise as they develop policies related to aging, and the scholars get to learn how things really operate in the federal government. My main fellowship project was to work for Health and Human Services in support of the

National Alzheimer's Project Act (NAPA). I was deeply impressed by the federal employees I met. They were idealistic, innovative, and smart; many had fancy PhDs and could easily make more money elsewhere. Instead, they hope to make a difference that will improve life in America. I think of them when I read about efforts to randomly amputate parts of the federal government, generally in the absence of information about what those groups do and what would happen if we stop them.

One major stumbling block is figuring out how to pay the people who provide care. Caring for people with dementia is hands-on hard work. Feeding someone, bathing her, getting rid of feces and urine—these are physical tasks that are tough to accomplish. Much of this care is provided by family members, but not all. There is an army of paid attendants who come into private homes to help out. Some come through agencies supported by Medicaid. Others come through agencies paid for by private funds, either out of pocket or partly covered by long-term care insurance. Many workers come through the informal market; they are hired without an agency, often through friends or relatives. They are a vulnerable group; 89 percent are women, the majority are women of color, and roughly a quarter were born in a foreign country.[15] Most earn close to or below minimum wage. Many have no paid sick leave. A worker with the flu knows her frail client could die from exposure to the disease, but has to choose between being paid or protecting her patient by staying away. Many receive no health insurance coverage; those able to buy health insurance through the Affordable Care Act are again in jeopardy under the current regime. Because of their low pay, they often rely on public assistance programs like Medicaid and food stamps to support their families.

Their work is often described as "unskilled," but you wouldn't think so if you tried it. Try to lift an adult who doesn't want to bathe into and out of a bathtub or help him with toileting. Many home care tasks cause injury. Because the work is hard and poorly paid, turnover rates are above 50 percent in many agencies.[16] For the demented person and his family, those constant personnel changes impose a real burden. Paranoia and fear are common in dementia. Introducing a new helper for an intimate task places a strain on worker and patient alike. At the same time, there is a substantial increase in the number of home care workers we'll need in the coming years to care for our aging population.

Home care agencies play a mixed role. Some are for profit, while others are nonprofit. Either way, an agency generally takes half the hourly fee, while the other half goes to the worker; the family or Medicaid may pay more than $20 an hour, but the worker takes home less than $10. Some localities require those on Medicaid to go through an agency to hire an aide. In this way the state provides oversight for quality of care, number of hours worked, and a complaint review process. If the worker fails to show, the agency finds a replacement.

Home care workers have played an active role in the movement to increase the minimum wage to $15 an hour. They had to work against many home care agencies, who clung to a ruling from years ago that exempted them from federal standards for minimum wage and overtime. That ruling was set aside in 2017, and at last these workers are covered by the same protections that fast-food workers and others count on. Home care workers have also pushed to unionize, as part of the effort to obtain benefits, training, and worker protections.

Not all families use agencies to find paid caregivers. Some want more control over who works in their home and how that work is done. Some are frustrated by agency rules that permit an elderly spouse to administer a complex medical regimen, but forbid a trained and paid caregiver to do the same. One family I met started out hiring through an agency, but then friends connected them to an informal network of aides from the former Soviet Union who were highly educated, often in the health care professions. When one would visit the old country or take a different job, he would find a replacement from within the community. In some of these arrangements, families pay above the going rate; the workers take home all the pay; and no one does burdensome paperwork. Though appealing, such arrangements often rely on undocumented workers and fail to report income, which are both common and quite illegal.

Hiring from outside an agency has liabilities for both employer and worker. A family could privately hire workers and pay them on the books, so they would receive Social Security and pay taxes, but only if they had documentation to work in the United States. Even for those eligible to work, many people break the law and skip the paperwork. A worker injured on such a job has little recourse; there is no worker's compensation, and no union to fight for better conditions, back pay, or benefits. Employers are at risk for failing to pay Social Security. Still, this shadow market is substantial, particularly in big cities with immigrants willing to accept jobs that documented workers shun.

Those who pay for long-term care using their own resources can drill a hole in even the deepest pockets. Tara Cortes is executive director at the Hartford Institute for Geriatric Nursing, a professor at the New York University Rory Meyers College of Nursing, and an internationally recognized expert in geriatric care. Even she had a lot to learn when her father, John Siegal, developed dementia. Her father was a remarkable man, an embodiment of the American dream. His parents emigrated from Poland as children and married at age sixteen. He was born in 1918 and played college football at Columbia. After college, the Chicago Bears recruited him, and he negotiated so he could attend dental school while on the team. He helped the Bears win three championships, and then switched to dentistry. When he died at ninety-seven, he was the oldest Chicago Bear.[17]

In old age, Siegal showed behavioral changes; he accused his wife of seventy years of renewing a relationship with a college sweetheart. His decline was slow and inexorable. He was on hospice for more than three years. Professor Cortes notes, "He had incredible insurance. He had Medicare, which paid for hospice. He had a Blue Cross supplement. And he had money from a settlement from the NFL, given his dementia, that gave him about $100,000 a year toward the end of his life. And even with all that, he went through an additional $80,000 yearly in those last few years."[18] Despite his exceptional access to long-term care funding, he nearly qualified for Medicaid at the end. His years of home care drained every asset.

Siegal's care was so expensive not because he went to a nursing home, but because his family kept him home, which they believed was the right thing to do. He had a whole team of workers, two for the day shift and two for the night, plus a separate aide to coordinate the team. He was big, as a pro football player would be, and not easily lifted, moved, or bathed. Several workers were devoted to Dr. Siegal and stayed on for years, but there was also considerable turnover and some uncaring, even insulting staff. Dr. Siegal had extensive insurance plus additional funds. He had an international expert in geriatric nursing to watch over his care. He didn't require Medicaid. His is the best-case scenario—and that should raise alarm bells. For most of us, things will fall far short of this picture, in terms of access, quality, and duration of care.

There appears to be a direct conflict between paying better wages to home care workers and offering more care at home for those with dementia. Yet we cannot ethically care for those with dementia when we fail to pay their caregivers a sustainable wage. A growing number of advocates are tackling the problem. Rick Surpin, a pioneer in the home care field, helped found the Cooperative Home Care Associates (CHCA) in 1985. Surpin is a dyed-in-the-wool lefty who was working thirty years ago for a community agency. His search for jobs for low-income women in the South Bronx evolved into the creation of a certified home care agency, cooperatively owned by workers. CHCA became the largest worker-owned coop in the United States. Its workers certainly need those jobs; 66 percent of trainees are single heads of households with minor children, 42 percent lack a high school diploma, and 56 percent had not worked in the year before joining CHCA.[19] CHCA's crucial innovation is that it forged an alliance between home care workers and their employers. Rather than pit worker and consumer against each other, Surpin and colleagues created a system where better care and better jobs benefited all parties. CHCA offers free training and rigorously screens those entering the program. After a period of probation, workers get health benefits, paid sick leave, and paid vacation. For longer-term employees, CHCA promises full-time hours for aides who want them. Workers sit on the board of directors and help set agency policy. Turnover is a fraction of industry rates. CHCA and its policy arm have played an important role in increasing pay and the quality of jobs not just within CHCA, but across the home care industry.[20]

MacArthur Foundation "genius" fellow Ai-jen Poo hoped to improve conditions for home care workers by founding the National Domestic Workers Alliance (NDWA) in 2007. Building on themes generated by Surpin and others, Poo aims to improve dignity both for workers and care recipients.[21] Successes have included the 2010 passage of the Domestic Workers' Bill of Rights, extending labor protections to domestic workers in New York State. She envisions a future in which families care for elderly and disabled members, sometimes with support from paid carers, and all enjoy the benefits of a cultural shift that values caregiving.

What would it take to provide better support at home? You'd have to start with the home itself. Is it accessible for a person who uses a wheelchair or has trouble walking? Are there steps to the house or inside? Are doors, including to the bathroom, wide enough to fit a wheelchair? Who could assess the home and recommend changes? Who would pay? In recent years there has been an increased focus on rehabilitating homes to help people age in place, with ramps, wheelchair lifts, bigger doors, and better lighting.[22] Putting money into rehabbing housing may help delay the far larger costs of a nursing home. Even putting in a bidet, or the more expensive bidet/toilet combination, may be one cost-effective way to stave off the nursing home.[23] Lots of elders with dementia hate to bathe; when you add that to incontinence, you have a bad situation. It's easier and safer to help someone keep clean using a bidet, and that might make all the difference in terms of how long care at home is manageable. Elevators are tough to install, but chair lifts can make some homes accessible. Some problems can't be fixed. A man may love the fifth-floor walk-up apartment he's lived in for sixty years, but if he can't walk, he can't get out in a fire.

If we look beyond the home to the neighborhood, an intriguing set of programs supports aging in place. These programs are not just for those with dementia, but are immensely helpful to them. A NORC, or naturally occurring retirement community, is a residential community not specifically designed for the elderly, but that has a majority of residents older than sixty. The first NORC was described in 1986 in a large apartment complex in New York City,[24] but today there are NORCs across the United States that connect elders with services for health and social interaction. NORCs tend to operate in urban areas for residents with economic vulnerability and functional impairment, and to rely on paid staff and government funding. A NORC can make all the difference between living at home or being forced into a nursing home. A social worker in an office off the lobby, an easy sign-up for transport to doctor's appointments, coordination with Meals on Wheels programs, outings, and exercise classes—these factors can be enough to keep an apartment building full of elders safely at home.

Similarly, the Village Movement got its start on Beacon Hill, an affluent section of Boston. There are now many Villages across the United States; these tend to serve clients who are financially more stable and have fewer functional impairments. Villages rely on volunteer service exchanges and are mainly financed by membership dues.[25] NORCs and Villages vary, but all facilitate access to services, enhance social interaction, and decrease social isolation. NORCs are more likely to link residents with government services, while a Village might provide a registry of discounted providers for home repair. Either may help organize grocery delivery for someone just home from the hospital, and both encourage a range of social activities. Neither NORCs nor Villages are designed for the demented elder. However, the services and social networks may help a person with mild or moderate dementia delay or avoid institutionalization, and can also help that person's spouse meet the challenge of supporting her at home.

For people whose impairments are more severe, there are adult day programs. A NORC may organize an outing to the local ball game, but the adult day program will offer help with feeding and toileting and will provide safeguards against wandering. These programs help family caregivers by offering respite and supporting their ability to hold down jobs and care for other family members.[26] Although a prime goal of adult day service programs has been to delay nursing home placement, research is unclear about whether they succeed in that specific aim.[27]

One major success story is the PACE program, or Program of All-Inclusive Care for the Elderly. These programs were pioneered at the On Lok senior center in San Francisco in 1971. The name means "peaceful, happy abode" in Cantonese.[28] To be eligible for PACE, a person must be disabled enough to meet criteria for nursing home placement, and also qualify for Medicare and Medicaid. PACE can provide the win-win we are looking for: The person stays happily and safely home, where he'd like to be, and the government need not fund expensive and unwanted nursing home care. PACE programs decrease the use of hospitals and nursing homes, and most participants improve or maintain function.[29] PACE saves money through lower cost preventive services like physical therapy, day centers, and primary care and social work visits. These allow participants to avoid expensive (and sometimes catastrophic) emergency room visits, hospital stays, or nursing home use. Because of its success in saving Medicaid dollars, the PACE model has been adapted to 114 sites and counting.[30]

Once a person moves into a nursing home, the chances of returning to the community dwindle. A program that fights against those odds is called Money Follows the Person. Acronym-loving bureaucrats (ALBs) refer to this program as MFP; it tackles barriers to returning home by coordinating community services and waiving Medicaid rules that prevent the use of long-term care funds outside a nursing home.[31] Funding through this program lasts a year, after which community programs are supposed to take over. The program has helped more than 40,000 people leave nursing homes to return to their communities.[32] Some of these elders later return to the nursing home, but many are grateful to have spent more time at home first.

An intriguing, even radical proposal for supporting elders at home is Medicaring Communities, the brainchild of Joanne Lynn, MD, director of the Center for Elder Care and Advanced Illness at the Altarum Institute. Dr. Lynn is a lesson in contrasts, a person of boundless energy whose academic expertise is frailty. She spent her childhood stomping around the mountains of West Virginia, eating the edible mushrooms and avoiding the poisonous ones. She is a highly regarded academic physician, especially for her role as a founder of the hospice movement. She got interested in hospice, though, to help support herself while she taught philosophy after medical school. As her career progressed, Lynn focused on frailty in older people, defined as unintended weight loss, exhaustion, weakness, and difficulty walking. Many people with dementia also have the multiple disabilities that constitute frailty. Her expertise now makes Lynn a cogent critic of hospice. As she notes, "Hospice is built on the idea you could promise to die on time. But if you're following a trajectory in which you can't know when you're going to die, then hospice is mis-constructed."[33] Lynn's frustration with the current supports available led her to devise Medicaring Communities, built around individualized treatment plans and local neighborhoods. "We pay for everything medical, but almost nothing for supportive services . . . We need a way to pay for your most important needs first . . . Housing, food, shelter, and someone to look after you. We now have large numbers of people with frailty and we haven't built the social arrangements to support them."[34]

Like its author, Medicaring is disarmingly straightforward, while proposing revolutionary differences in the way care is provided. It bands together proven programs, including PACE, but sets them within a geographic neighborhood. Lynn argues that anchoring programs in a neighborhood makes sense; clinicians visiting multiple local patients waste less time and money by minimizing commuting. But most programs don't operate this way. There is a belief that all providers must serve all communities, or poorer neighborhoods won't get equal service. While it's true poor communities often are overlooked, there is little evidence they do better when providers are spread out across a large region. Lynn argues that unless you can focus and coordinate services within a neighborhood, the endeavor of helping people stay in their homes will fall apart. "You can't care for a dementia patient at home if you have no way to get food into the home, no way to get to a doctor's appointment, and no doctor will go see them."[35] Lynn provides compelling data to show that Medicaring can help keep frail elders out of the hospital by offering better basic supports, and save enough money to pay for them by cutting back on expensive, unhelpful medical interventions.[36] She hopes to start demonstration projects, but so far has not found the funding. If she is right, Medicaring offers a way to provide the care that people want, at home, safely, for lower costs. That is the recipe we are looking for.

We could learn a lot by looking at how other developed nations care for frail and demented elders. *The American Health Care Paradox* by Elizabeth Bradley and Lauren Taylor documents that good health results don't come only from expenditures on traditional medical care.[37] Other developed nations have long had better health outcomes than the United States, and this sad fact has puzzled many, particularly since the U.S. spends far more than any other nation on medical care. The secret is that we spend less on social services. If you add what is spent on medical care to what is spent on social services, we are in the middle of developed nations, which corresponds to our middling health results. Spending on social services makes a huge difference. The kind of services Lynn proposes with Medicaring—meals, transportation, social work visits—are exactly the services that produce better health in other developed nations.

Getting America to offer better social support services is a heavy lift. We have a much easier time paying for expensive technology, especially expensive medical technology. We don't like "halfway technology" that just supports someone with disability. We like a *fix*. Problem is, frail elders with dementia don't have something that can be fixed. Support is exactly what they need. We think we can't afford that support. That's partly because we've already spent our money on other things, including unhelpful medical interventions.

The number of people in nursing homes is dropping and the number of nursing home beds is shrinking, due to nursing home closure and the conversion of beds to better-reimbursed short-term care. Medicaid cuts are constantly threatened, and patients in nursing homes are the ones most threatened by those cuts. While programs are popping up around the country to pay for care that helps elders with dementia stay home as long as possible, those programs are unevenly distributed. It is a great deal easier to form a NORC in an urban setting, with a social worker or primary care clinic right in the building, than it is in suburbia or in farm country. For communities with less well funded and organized public health infrastructure, life with dementia can be even more hazardous and lonely. Those who can will fall back on family, faith communities, and neighbors, and sometimes that is enough. Sometimes it just isn't. A significant portion of those eighty-five and older live alone. Many have no relatives to provide assistance.

As a nation, we don't have a viable plan to pay for dementia care. People go without help that would be useful because we spend our money on things that don't improve quality or quantity of life. As Joanne Lynn notes, anyone over sixty-five can get an expensive hospital stay paid for, but they run into a lot of trouble getting help to prevent that hospitalization. Many good people are wrestling with this problem. But right now we have a big ugly hole in our health care policy. The problem of paying for dementia care is heading like a meteor toward the children of the baby boom generation. We need to fix this, and soon. The current administration isn't even looking at the problem, but that won't make it go away.

Chapter 10

Laborers of Love

M oney fixes some problems, but not all. Mrs. S lives in an elegant apartment in a grand old building on the Upper West Side of Manhattan. Mrs. S is tiny and exceedingly determined. She is funny and frank. She is a painter; her home is painterly. Light flows in from three sides and the colors are deep and jewel-like. But caring for her late husband when he had dementia was not easy for Mrs. S. Thinking back on her marriage, Mrs. S told me, "We managed not to get along for sixty years, we never agreed on anything, but it was also good in certain ways."[1]As he entered his eighties, Mr. S started to change for the worse, and Mrs. S grew increasingly frustrated by her inability to get his doctor to listen to her and intervene. Mr. S had trouble in the past with his prostate and had seen a urologist, but refused to go back, even though he developed incontinence. "He would not get help, he would not wear a diaper. But he wouldn't go just anywhere—he would walk into the kitchen and pee on the floor. Since he didn't do it in the living room he seemed to have some control, but how much? What was happening? . . . At a certain point I refused to go out with him because I was afraid of what would happen."

Mr. S's personality changed as well. Though their marriage always included friction, the tone shifted. He swore at Mrs. S—he had never done that before. "I would ask him something and he'd come back with, 'Oh, go away. You're a fucking pain in the ass.'" He pushed her and physically threatened her. Mr. S would not act this way with everyone—he retained the capacity to behave appropriately with visitors and people he knew less well, reserving his abuse for his wife of nearly sixty years. He had a strong will and began to insist on irrational things. He would want to leave the apartment late at night, including in the winter. He would claim he was going on a trip and needed to keep $200 in his pants pockets at all times, "for expenses." But he was incontinent, and so the bills were washed again and again, demonstrating the sturdiness of the paper on which they were printed, if not of their owner. His sleep-wake cycles changed and he was awake for hours at night.

When Mr. and Mrs. S had become empty nesters, they sold their family apartment and moved to a smaller two-bedroom, planning to use the difference to help fund their retirement. But as Mr. S's condition deteriorated, his incontinence and late-night demands meant Mrs. S needed help at night. An aide slept in the tiny second bedroom. Mrs. S, in her eighties, could not share a wet bed with her husband; she slept on the living room couch. This was not a happy long-term solution, although it is a common arrangement for elderly partners of people with dementia. Mrs. S consulted her adult children and figured out what she could afford. She did not consult Mr. S, who was once highly astute with finances. She sold her apartment and moved again, to a three-bedroom. It's not what she had hoped for, but she was glad she was still able to make this change. Goodbye, empty nesting. Goodbye, nest egg. Now there would be separate bedrooms for Mr. S, Mrs. S, and an aide.

Architecture made a difference in Mrs. S's efforts to care for her husband. If you want to age in place, you should consider where you, an impaired spouse, and a helper will all sleep. Downsizing has a huge appeal in an expensive city like New York, but what seems like a prudent financial move at one point may create burdens later. And the number of bedrooms wasn't the only issue. The offices of some of Mr. S's doctors were in brownstones. The aide and Mrs. S would have to get his walker, later his wheelchair, down the steps, push a buzzer, get through the door to push another buzzer, and then maneuver Mr. S and his devices into a cramped hall. It was dangerous and unpleasant all around.

Mrs. S put together a team of helpers. The costs were large, but were partly defrayed by a long-term care insurance policy that covered a portion of the in-home care. Mrs. S paid for the remaining substantial costs out of pocket. For the last four months of his life, Mr. S had round-the-clock care, with people doing different shifts. The S family was lucky. For most Americans, who neither have sufficient private resources nor Medicaid, this level of care is an impossibility.

Mrs. S credits her primary helper, Ms. M, for pulling her through those final months. The bonds of affection between these two women are poignant and clear. Ms. M had previously worked for a different family in their old apartment building. She came to the S family with little formal training in health care, but great natural talent. Over the course of time, as an astute observer, Ms. M learned what helped and harmed her efforts to care for Mr. S. It wasn't easy, and not every helper stayed the course. He would pull hair, swear, push, and yell, particularly when aides tried to bathe him—he was afraid of falling and became especially aggressive when afraid. He would also become aggressive if told no, so Ms. M learned not to tell him no. He became sensitive to noise and would tell her not to speak. She knew then that he would blow up if she spoke, so she did not. When he started to get angry, his face would change and she learned to leave him alone for a bit. Asked how she was able to work so well with Mr. S, she answered, "Compassion. I think that [dementia] may be my future and I would like to be treated well. I feel for him a lot. My father also had the same disease."

I asked Mrs. S if she ever considered putting her husband into a nursing facility as his behavior became more difficult. She had thought about it, but they had a very brief, very bad experience that set her against nursing homes. When they were getting set to move to the larger apartment, they arranged for Mr. S and an aide to stay at a local facility for a few days, while the old place was packed up and the new one assembled. But when they arrived on a Sunday evening, no one had heard of them—no bed was ready, and there was no agreement that the aide could stay in Mr. S's room. The staff was disorganized and unhelpful. Mr. S also had cancer, and soon after that, he began to decline more quickly. Mrs. S decided that a nursing home was not in his future: "We can't do that to him."

Mr. and Mrs. S appear not to have received sound medical advice, despite living in Manhattan, surrounded by premier medical institutions. This is not uncommon. Good dementia care requires a team, but American medicine can devolve into individual specialists from different networks who never communicate, never integrate, and never see the big picture. Each doctor sees the patient as a kidney or an ear or whatever, with a bit of skin and some other stuff around it, but not as a human who has multiple problems, many of which are not even medical. Standards for dementia care and assessment have changed greatly in the last decade. Many doctors only recognize dementia in the bed-bound final phase, but not in those with moderate symptoms. Everywhere she turned, Mrs. S faced barriers and frustrations. Mr. S's main doctor was a cardiologist; Mrs. S could not engage him in any discussion of Mr. S's changing behavior. Like a bad waiter in a busy restaurant, he basically told her, "That's not my table."

After considerable time, once Mr. S was already incontinent and had greatly diminished cognitive capacity, the cardiologist referred him to a psychiatrist—not a neurologist. Usually a neurologist takes the lead in assessing dementia, but there are many psychiatrists, especially geriatric psychiatrists, who provide skillful care for dementia patients and coordinate with other specialists for whatever help is needed. Best of all might be a geriatrician, who has the skills to view older patients in the context of multiple illnesses, and who is more likely to partner with a social worker to help families navigate health care and benefit issues. The best care for a man like Mr. S—with both behavioral and cognitive symptoms—involves an integrated team working in collaboration. My institution, Montefiore, sponsors the Center for the Aging Brain with coordinated care from multiple professionals, and other hospitals have similar approaches. Still, far too few people get the kind of thorough, thoughtful, competent care that a patient with dementia deserves. Mrs. S describes the psychiatrist Mr. S ended up seeing as "a very nice person, but he wasn't forceful." Mr. S was a highly intelligent man, and retained the capacity to be socially appropriate at his appointments. The doctor told Mrs. S that since her husband was not verbally abusive to him, he was unable to help her with that. He had no advice on what Mrs. S, who is less than five feet tall, should do when Mr. S would try to push past her to get out of the apartment at night. The psychiatrist either did not know or didn't care that his dapper older patient habitually peed on the kitchen floor. As far as Mrs. S could tell, the psychiatrist and Mr. S mostly discussed local restaurants. The doctor did not invite Mrs. S to join a discussion with him and her husband. He shared with Mrs. S no diagnosis, no medications, no assessment of Mr. S's altered emotional or cognitive status, no treatment options, and no suggestions on how Mrs. S should cope. Nor did he refer to a professional who could do any of this. As a psychiatrist, I am shamed by this story. Admittedly, I know the story only from the perspective of the grieving Mrs. S. Nonetheless, the details are plausible. A physician cannot heal every patient. But any practitioner should strive to make a diagnosis and a plan, or refer to someone who can.

Then Mr. S fell, whacked his head, and was referred to a neurologist for the first time. Months after that, as the injury was healing, the neurologist noted in passing that Mr. S had dementia—that was the first time any doctor used this word. It was years after Mrs. S had noticed and reported to other physicians the changes in Mr. S. To this day Mrs. S doesn't know what type of dementia her husband had. He retained some aspects of memory right up until the end—he could direct Ms. M back to the new apartment when she had trouble finding the way but had marked changes in mood, personality, executive function, and judgment. Mrs. S was not surprised by the diagnosis; she had been saying for ages that something was wrong, and finally his doctors agreed. When asked what she most would have wanted to make her caregiving easier, she said, "A doctor who listens to the family, because after all they're the ones who see things happen. A doctor who respects the observer." Such a modest request. Mr. and Mrs. S should never have gone without this simple form of respect.

Hospice was the one bright spot for this family. After a time it became clear that Mr. S would succumb to his collection of illnesses—cancer, dementia, cardiac disease, and others—and hospice was called in. Mrs. S can't say enough positive things about their experience. "They were a great help! I am never going to forget that. We had a great nurse . . . She stayed with him for three nights at the end. She sat with him and she prayed . . . They really are terrific. If you call them in the middle of the night, they'll have somebody there."

The end game is never easy. I asked Mrs. S what care she might want if she were old, frail, and perhaps demented. She said, "I'd want to die." She's quite serious. She has looked into the aid in dying movement, into what's on offer in Oregon and California and Switzerland. She is in no hurry, but her experience as a caregiver left her troubled. She didn't like the role she was in, and she didn't like seeing Mr. S become unrecognizable. Nor would she like her children or anyone else to have to take on the role she had. Money helps with some things, but nothing removes the sting of watching a loved one become someone you don't know.

To study the impact on caregivers of people with dementia is to contemplate the prospect of bad things happening to good people. Caregivers suffer for the pains they take to support family members. They have worse health outcomes than their peers, including increased rates of depression and heart disease.[2] They don't live as long as similar people who did not care for a demented family member at home.[3] If they give up outside work to be a caregiver, they will have a lower income, less money saved for retirement, less money to expect from Social Security, and fewer resources to call upon when they themselves are older and perhaps disabled.[4] Since dementia runs in families, those caring for parents with dementia are more likely than others to also get dementia.

These findings are not new; they have been demonstrated in multiple studies over many years. Even so, many caregivers would not give up their efforts—it is enormously important to them to support a loved one at home. Like Mrs. S, they just can't send someone they care about to an institution. The act of caregiving has produced some remarkable narratives, personal stories that clarify the experience in a way that data cannot. John Bayley, the husband of Iris Murdoch, offered through his memoirs a moving account of a caregiver who was both loving and nearly overwhelmed by the job.[5] Both Bayley and Murdoch were Oxford professors. Murdoch's fiery intellect made her a successful novelist as well as an Oxford don in philosophy. But late in life, she inadvertently broadcast her cognitive decline in an ill-fated television interview. Her failing memory blocked her from answering basic questions; she stared blankly at the camera until the host stopped the interview in consternation.

Murdoch and Bayley's decades together featured unbelievably high standards for intellectual discourse, surrounded as they were by the cream of the English intelligentsia. Standards for domestic hygiene, even when they were young and healthy, were rather looser. Bayley summarizes the approach to household cleanliness as befits a great scholar of English literature, by quoting Keats: "But where the dead leaf fell, there did it rest." The reality was less poetic: Photographs and descriptions of their home show stacks of unwashed dishes, piles of papers on the stairs, and conditions generally that would make a social worker blanch. Despite clutter and chaos, Bayley offered a portrait of a loving home as Murdoch became increasingly impaired and her devoted husband aged beside her. They journeyed together into a land created by dementia. As Bayley writes:

> Every day, we are physically closer; and Iris's little "mouse cry," as I think of it, signifying loneliness in the next room, the wish to be back beside me, seems less and less forlorn, more simple, more natural. She is not sailing into the dark:

The voyage is over, and under the dark escort of Alzheimer's,
she has arrived somewhere. So have I.[6]

Bayley showed us the merging of caregiver and receiver, aging together in the way they chose and desired. It was a way not without
difficulties, nor a way everyone might choose, but it was their way, and
it just suited.

Different caregivers face different challenges. George Hodgman, in
Bettyville: A Memoir,[7] describes his return to the dwindling Missouri
town of his childhood to care for his widowed mother as dementia and
other illnesses converge in her old age. Like many adult children caring for a demented parent, Hodgman is struck by the sense of taboo,
of the impossibility of telling his mother what shoes to wear, when to
sleep and to eat. Who has put him in charge? Certainly not his mother!
And yet she can no longer cope alone, and Hodgman must do his best
to help, without forcing her to recognize her dependence or express the
gratitude that recognition might inspire.

Many researchers focus on the plight of caregivers. What can be
done to ease the burden, to support them so they are not wounded by
their good work? There are a range of motives behind this concern.
There is an ethical obligation to honor and support those who do the
important work of caring for people with dementia at home—their
efforts make it possible to honor the wishes of people with dementia.
Still, it is not lost on government funding agencies that when caregivers burn out, they are more likely to end up institutionalizing their
family member. Supporting the family could be the path to big savings in nursing home costs. Delaying institutionalization even by a
year can mean saving tens of thousands of dollars per person.

One of the great experts on caregivers is Carol Levine. She got into this line of work, literally, by accident. She and her husband were driving together back in 1990 and were in a terrible car crash. She walked away, but he was severely disabled until his death, seventeen years later.[8] After the accident, Howard Levine was in a coma for four months, and then went to a rehab facility after he finally regained consciousness. Only there, six months after the crash, did Carol Levine first hear from a young physician that her husband was unlikely to recover anything like his former level of physical ability. Prior to that she had been given a message of absurd, unfounded optimism ("He's going to walk out of here!"), mostly from the neurosurgeon who operated on him. Bringing her husband home meant acquiring a whole new skill set, from completing mountains of paperwork to advocating for additional services or insisting that a health professional look again at a set of symptoms and help find a solution. Her husband came home with undiagnosed depression and sleep apnea, overlooked by the medical team as they focused on more immediately threatening issues. Sorting out his medical illnesses and getting appropriate treatment was difficult, but over time she got it done.

What proved much harder was coping with some of the comments and attitudes from "helping" professionals, many of them women. When faced with any difficulty in the medical care system, she was told the problem was her attitude. A nurse at the rehab facility said, "If you were a good wife, you would sleep on the floor." One social worker advised her to just quit her job and go on Medicaid. For emphasis, she added, "Your life is over. Get used to it." Stunned at first, Levine began to fight back. "I got a little tougher and started to be more assertive. I was learning about the system and about my place in it and stiffening my spine. I began to say no one can do this to us."[9]

Levine realized she couldn't possibly be the only one in her situation and began to study caregivers. She didn't quit her job and go on

Medicaid. Instead, soon after the social worker's helpful suggestion, she won a MacArthur Foundation "genius" award to carry out her work. For the last twenty years Levine has directed the Families and Health Care project at the United Hospital Fund. Her wealth of experience has produced many insights. One is that procedures that require advanced training when performed in hospitals by health care professionals are often handed off to family members with almost no training to do in an unsupervised home setting. This is not a good plan, and better training for family members would help prevent both distress and bad outcomes for the disabled family member. And reasonable limits to expectations of what a family member can do would also help.

Another insight is that even with better training and supervision, there is a profound psychological disparity between a uniformed health professional's working intimately with a stranger's body and a family member's working with a loved one. There is all the difference in the world between a nurse changing a diaper on an adult patient in the ICU and an adult son changing his mother's diaper in the home where he grew up. As Levine notes, "there is a failure to understand from the professional side that there's an emotional component to doing these things—even the things you can do—without feeling you are doing something horribly wrong." In general, the medical system has done a shabby job of preparing family carers for either the technical or psychological aspects of the role.

She also learned that providing care is not the hardest part of being a caregiver. Coping with the medical system, including its many harassed and unsympathetic representatives, was for her the worst part. The mountains of forms from insurance programs, the endless calls, the petitioning to receive benefits one has paid for, the scheduling of visits to and from various professionals—"the lack of empathy or professionalism or human consciousness about doing a job that's not just fixing the TV"—they are all excruciating.

No one knows better that it's tough to be a family caregiver, but Levine would not have bypassed her experience. It was important to her to keep her husband, Howard, at home all those years, and to keep him integrated as much as possible into the lives of their children. Though he is gone now, he still matters to her and to them. She feels lucky she was able to use what she learned to help others, and that in doing so she found a new purpose in her life, in a way that made a difference to her. "To take one's personal experience and try to expand it to a social problem was my way of making meaning out of it all. That's important for people. It's not to make you feel better. It makes the pieces fit together."

Levine points out that "bioethics has done families a disservice by focusing solely on the individual autonomy of the patient. That's a prime value, but not the only value. Families enter into the space of caregiving in a way that bears consideration and bears as much respect as the individual autonomy of the patient."[10] Helping people with disabilities live at home, receiving the support they need without entering an institution, is an important step toward more ethical health policies. What we've done less well as a society is to consider how we will also support those who, paid or unpaid, make the choice to stay home possible. There are those who bemoan the lack of responsibility in families today, claiming there would be no need for expensive government programs if families took care of their own as they ought. This line of reasoning ignores the well-documented fact that the vast majority of care, certainly for those with dementia, is provided by family members without compensation. It also fails to acknowledge that dementia is a disease of aging. Large numbers of people with dementia have outlived their relatives—there is no family left to blame.

Bioethics has had relatively little to say on this issue of how we should balance our support for those with disabilities with the values and needs of those who provide that support.[11]

Mary Mittelman, an epidemiologist and professor in the Department of Psychiatry at New York University, is prominent among the scholars working to offer better support to family caregivers. If you met Mittelman on a boat in the Arabian Sea, you would still know immediately that she is a New Yorker. She has a slight New York accent, but it is more that she is fast-talking, lively, genial, and very candid. She is also funny, and more than a little exasperated by what is generally viewed as valuable in research on dementia. Mittelman is best known for her work in designing, implementing, and evaluating a deceptively simple and highly effective counseling intervention to support family caregivers.[12] The program consists of some counseling sessions for the main caregiver and other family members, a support group, and the option for backup phone calls and advice as needed. She notes, "We don't have our act together in terms of policy . . . We put bazillions of dollars into millions of efforts to find the drug that is going to prevent dementia."[13] As Mittelman notes, she is of an age such that this long-off cure is not going to save her. She is frustrated that the caregiver intervention she has worked on for years is suddenly attracting more attention—but not for the reasons she would prefer. "Our paper showed that if Minnesota made the intervention available to the whole state, it would save them $998 million a year. I am glad something talks, but I am offended that it's not that these people might be less stressed, less depressed, and physically healthier; that's not what's important."[14] What appears to be important is that compared with a matched set of families without the intervention, the study subjects delayed admitting their family member to a nursing facility by a significant period, even for those with advanced dementia.

Taking care of the carers meant they could keep their job longer, and that means a whopping potential savings for Minnesota and the rest of the country.

When pressed to say what should be different in our approach to dementia, Mittelman answers that well-designed psychosocial interventions should be a part of most, if not all, treatment plans. Mittelman does not spare her colleagues in the field. She finds many studies sloppily designed and with too few subjects to reach a valid conclusion. For her, this work is critically important. She wants to see more funding, higher research standards, more innovations, and more progress. Like many dementia researchers, Mittelman had a family member—her mother—with the disease. She wishes her late mother could have had better care, and that she herself had had better guidance in providing it. When she introduces the caregiver intervention to new groups, she often tells them about what it was like when her mother had advanced dementia. Back then Mittelman had two small children, a husband who didn't cook, and a full-time job. Her father told her, "It's your time to care for her." She had no idea how to do that, what it would mean, how to get started, or how to handle her other responsibilities. Mittelman hopes her groundwork will make it possible for others to provide high-quality loving care for a parent with dementia.

There are caregivers who get support from some truly excellent programs, and there are caregivers who don't get anywhere near enough support. Sometimes the same people fall into both categories. Caring-Kind, which used to be the New York branch of the Alzheimer's Association, focuses on providing help for caregivers. They offer support groups for people at different stages of dementia, including in the earliest phases, and other groups for caregivers. I sat in on such a meeting and came away impressed with the strength and compassion of the participants and also the magnitude of their responsibilities. The members were exuberantly enthusiastic about the skill of their facilitator, Sharon Shaw, an experienced clinical social worker. A few had been in other support groups with weak facilitators, and the experience was so bad it *increased* the caregivers' sense of stress. They praised Sharon for her skill in knowing just what any member was feeling or might need. She took that compliment as an opportunity to applaud the attendees for how well they had learned to read one another, and said that was why the group was so effective and supportive. It was a deft intervention. I had to agree that Sharon's knowledge and warmth came shining through. She is an excellent facilitator.

Mostly, participants talked about how isolating it can be to care for someone with dementia. Friends fall away. The assignment is never over. It may be the middle of the night, but you are still awake because your spouse is awake, or cleaning up the bathroom because he can't use it without accidents. The group left them feeling less alone. There were also practical benefits. They'd learn from another member about a trick to calm agitation, or a new medicine or a side effect. They were learning, they weren't alone, and their work as caregivers was understood and appreciated.

They all faced different challenges. Memory issues per se were not their biggest problem. One woman's husband would periodically fail to recognize her. Then he'd become enraged and call the police.

"He was the sweetest man. Now he has behavioral issues. When he doesn't believe I belong in the house, there's no reasoning with him. The police came out twice. He said, 'Get her out of here!' The first time there were four of them. Two had family members with Alzheimer's disease and they were very familiar. Two went into the other room with my husband. I stayed sobbing in the living room. Fifteen minutes later they all come back and he says, 'Let's go for a drink!' Like nothing ever happened."[15]

After a pause, another group member gently asked, "What do you do when he gets agitated like that?" She answered, "Seroquel [an antipsychotic medication]." Another group member said, "For you or him?" They all laughed. They'd all been there.

For another member, the hardest thing was repetition. His wife would get into a loop in which she repeated the same few sentences over and over for hours, sometimes varying the order, as part of an imaginary conversation. She'd ask after herself by her maiden name, and after a fellow from her village in the old country. If she looked in the mirror, she might take on different parts of the conversation. She was always caught in the same whirlpool, the same phrases that went nowhere. To call it repetition didn't capture how awful this was to watch. The broken networks of her brain made a cage; she couldn't get out and he couldn't get in.

Outside of the group, it's not possible to speak of these things. People don't want to hear. Old friends and family may ask how the person with dementia is doing. Almost no one asks how the caregiver is doing. In the group, they ask and can honestly answer. It's a lifeline.

Whether a caregiver is paid or not, a person with dementia cannot stay home without backup once the disease progresses past a certain point. Consider Mrs. C, a sweet and talkative woman with moderate dementia. She had almost every known risk factor, including very limited formal education; though she could barely read, she was passed along to eighth grade and then dropped out, mostly because she was so "wild." In her teens she fell from a rooftop while sniffing glue. She sustained massive trauma to every part of her body, including her head, leaving her with traumatic brain injury. She abstains now, but had a long history of abusing alcohol. She has had severe depression, as well as cardiovascular disease and diabetes, the latter of which left her with an amputated leg. Right now, she stays in her own apartment; she waited years for this housing, which is accessible, with an elevator. She has a helper, supported by Medicaid, who comes in for several hours on weekdays. She does a great job, making sure Mrs. C is okay, preparing meals, cleaning, and helping her get set for the day. Mrs. C's sleep-wake cycle is a mess, but she knows that if she wakes up and it is dark out, she should stay home and watch TV until her helper arrives in the morning. Her small apartment is spotless and homey. She has big pillows set up on the floor, where she can comfortably watch TV despite her amputation. She has a framed photo of J.Lo (revered in the Bronx as a local goddess) on the windowsill. A motorized scooter helps her get out to the grocery store and the local park. For now, she has what she needs.

Without a caregiver, living on your own with dementia is dangerous, for you and for those around you. For another one of Dr. Ceide's patients, the risks were just too great. Mrs. D was ninety-five, growing old alone with increasingly severe cognitive deficits. Concerned social workers had been tracking her situation, actively trying and failing to improve her living condition for more than a year. There was one member of her extended family left in the local area, but as Mrs. D became more paranoid, she stopped letting that person into the apartment. Then she stopped letting anyone in. But Dr. Ceide has a special talent for communication. People who trust no one trust her. Mrs. D permitted Dr. Ceide to slip in through the cracked open door. Mrs. D was quite thin—she was no longer adequately feeding herself. Her home was beyond filthy, with piles of old paper and garbage narrowing every space; something awful was smeared on a wall. Mrs. D herself was filthy. The bathtub was full of trash, and it was unclear if the plumbing still worked. She had boarded up the living room windows because of her paranoia. She kept several pigeons in an old laundry basket in the living room. She had refused many times to let a home attendant into her apartment to clean or care for her. She had a son, but he lived a thousand miles away, and was in his seventies and also ill. The situation was untenable. It was no longer safe for Mrs. D to live on her own, and had not been for some time. It was not safe for the other people in the building to have a neighbor live this way. After careful negotiations with Mrs. D, the distant son, the caseworkers, the local relative, and the emergency room, Dr. Ceide called 911. She accompanied Mrs. D to the emergency room, comforting her and making sure that no one frightened her or treated her roughly. They found a nursing home. Mrs. D was unhappy to leave her apartment, but there was no way around it. At a certain point, dementia and isolation are a fatal combination. Health professionals like Dr. Ceide go out of their way to honor autonomy. They work hard to find ways to support someone at home if that's what they want. But they must also determine when the dignity of freedom decays into misery and neglect. It is still possible today to uncover people living with dementia much as Dorothea Dix found the woman out in the cold. We have learned a great deal in two hundred years, but we have not perfected the art of balancing freedom and safety, of getting the right care to people who need it.

The experience of being a caregiver is always hard, but it's not always bad. There's a difference. Mrs. T cherishes her experience caring for her late husband. When she first met R through mutual friends, she had been widowed only a few months. His wife had died at almost the same time as her husband. They had dinner with friends, and afterward, he volunteered to walk her the few blocks home. The next day he sent flowers. They knew right away they were right for each other, but they waited for a bit more than a year to get married.

They both had kids but all were adults in their own right. "It was very romantic," she says, smiling hugely.[16] Just when things had looked bleakest, just when their expectations were lowest, they found love and a happy marriage. Things went along well for more than twenty years. They were social. They saw their friends, their children, and the multiplying grandchildren. They felt lucky. They were.

Then R started to have trouble at work. His son was his partner and there were terrible strains between them. R's judgment became erratic and the business was affected. Mrs. T knew something was wrong but she didn't know what. R remained cheerful with all their friends; he was always kind to her, the same old person. Nonetheless they went to see a neurologist at a prestigious hospital. The son encouraged this examination; R was unaware that anything was wrong. The doctor confirmed there was substantial memory loss. Mrs. T didn't care for this doctor. "He was awful! So unempathic!" They switched doctors, but R continued to decline, holding on to his sunny personality but losing his ability to work, judge, or make decisions. Then he fell and hurt his arm, giving him severe pain. "That was the beginning of the end. After the fall, he turned yellow. My prior husband had died of pancreatic cancer and I knew this was it again, before any of the tests came back."[17]

After that, things happened quickly. Mrs. T moved her husband out of the bedroom because he was up all night and she couldn't sleep. She got more help until she had a team of three men around the clock for the last few months. She took many of her meals with them as R got weaker. She became very close to them; she knew all about their private lives, becoming a kind of honorary grandmother. While I interviewed her, one of them dropped by to say hello. While R was still aware, he preferred Mrs. T to change his diaper; he was embarrassed to have the male helpers do it. She didn't mind; she was happy to do

206 · DEMENTIA REIMAGINED

what she could for him. "At the end, he didn't know." It didn't matter then who changed his diaper.

Mrs. T saw the combination of dementia and cancer as a kind of blessing. The dementia meant R was not frightened of the cancer; he couldn't retain the information that he had it. And it was a blessing he had the cancer because that set a limit on his dementia and how long he would suffer. Mrs. T sees a lot of things as blessings. She is a spectacularly resilient and optimistic person. Though it was so hard, she doesn't feel she suffered in caring for her husband, though this was the second time she was widowed. She is grateful for the support she received from her family. Her daughter was "her rock," her children and R's stepped up, her helpers really dedicated themselves. She also managed to find some great programs in her community. She went with R to The Memory Tree, a New York City program for people with memory loss and their families. They did chair yoga and an art appreciation class. R would never have agreed to go to a program if he knew it was for people with dementia, but with his wife by his side, he thought it must be okay. For her it was wonderful to be able to be in a group and not to have to explain any lapses, but just enjoy the outing and the companionship. Mrs. T had a great team, and a large, loving, and supportive family, and the program still made a big difference.

I asked Mrs. T what kind of care she would want if she were frail and demented, and she immediately said she'd like to be in a home. I misunderstood her and said, "You'd like to be at home?" She clarified: "No. I'd like to be in a nursing home. I like all the activities. It's not so lonely. I like to be around people. And I'd hate for my children to be stuck caring for me." I heard this response more than once. Many caregivers wouldn't put their loved one in a nursing home, but they didn't object to being in one themselves. They like the sociability of communal living; they fear isolation more than institutionalization, especially if they find the right institutional setting. They also think the burden of caregiving was more than they could impose on someone they loved.

D ecisions about caregiving hit different families differently. In 2013, J was president of a think tank, with a glamorous life. She was careful about her diet and an avid yoga practitioner. And then, in her early fifties, she developed odd symptoms in rapid succession. These turned out to be frontotemporal dementia. Her husband, D, describes how her illness unfolded:[18]

> We both thought [J] was depressed. She was very worried about my health—I had a recurrence of cancer. That was very difficult for her, more difficult at the time than it was for me. I noticed odd behavior that fall, out of character . . . shopping for things she didn't need, that kind of thing. But the first day I was *really* scared was when we got back from a trip, late on a Tuesday evening. It became clear as we got into the house that [J] had missed an event for work that afternoon. She said, "I'll go tomorrow." I said, "No, today is Tuesday, the event was today—you can't go tomorrow." And she couldn't get over that today was Tuesday and she couldn't go tomorrow. She couldn't understand why. We went around and around on this. And I couldn't understand what was happening—why did she not understand? This is a woman who was running a think tank. Very scary . . . That was January. By March everything was settled.

"Settled" in this case meant that J's diagnosis of frontotemporal dementia was crystal clear. There were no effective treatments. She was suddenly and significantly disabled. Within months, J could not be left alone in the house. Her sleep-wake cycles went haywire. J was so restless at night that D took to sleeping on the couch, but this was no good. He had cancer, he had a full-time job, and he needed sleep. J, once "the most considerate person in the world," could no longer retain the information that she should try to keep quiet in the middle of the night. She was never malicious; she had simply lost the ability to grasp the impact of her actions.

J deteriorated rapidly. She had a scary hospitalization due to problems with her immune system. When she came home, helpers came to care for her, but they were bewildered. J was still in her fifties, as is common for those with frontotemporal dementia. She didn't look sick, though she had just spent months gravely ill in a hospital. It was hard for them to figure out what the problem was and how to help, and J couldn't clarify. She lost all executive function, meaning she couldn't plan and implement a series of actions to get to even a simple goal. She couldn't dress herself; she couldn't plan to put on underwear before pants, pants before shoes. She couldn't make a sandwich. She couldn't be left alone with a stove, or a door that led out to the great city. She could move quickly but had no judgment. She was like a toddler, except that everyone recognizes a toddler should not be on the street by herself, while J looked like any other adult. D despaired. He made a decision, a difficult one. J was admitted to a nursing home.

When D talks about this, you can hear his ambivalence. He doesn't want you to feel sorry for him. He doesn't mention his recurrent cancer as a factor. He states that another person might not have made this choice, and maybe there were additional steps he could have taken, ones he didn't see at the time. He could have quit his job—though the job was keeping him sane. He could have moved to a separate apartment, but that would have been weird, too. He made the decision he made with the information he had, and it was the right decision for them. It was still tough. He feels the stigma of sending a loved one to a nursing home. He needed to keep J safe. He could no longer do it at home. She had excellent care, even as she became increasingly frail and lost weight, as is typical of the late stage of dementia. She died after two years. The director of the nursing home noted that J was the first person he'd admitted, in decades of working there, who was younger than he was.

Many of us are deeply ambivalent about nursing homes. Some people need them—there really is no other setting that will work for their level of disability. And some people would rather be with other people than home alone (or nearly alone). They find the thought of being on their own, aged and disabled, lonely. They don't want their family to bear the burden of caregiving or managing a team of caregivers. Some nursing homes are warm and comforting places of refuge for those who live there, and they work really hard to be that way. But there are too few that meet this goal. Many families dread placing a relative in a home. Despite Mr. S's insults and hair-pulling, Mrs. S could not bring herself to do it. Other people won't put their spouse in a nursing home but would be fine with that for themselves. High-quality care, tailor-made for someone you love or even for you, might happen at your house, but maybe not. To get it right, we're going to have to learn some flexibility and open our minds to finding out what works.

Many people want to stay home as long as possible. The more help is available and the more a person accepts it, the longer that is feasible. Too fierce an insistence on independence can result in disaster. Some symptoms are harder to manage at home; families are often overwhelmed by paranoia, incontinence, disrupted sleep-wake cycles, agitation, and wandering. We can't get dementia care right by only asking the person what she would like. Someone has to provide that care. We have to create a system that provides the help both people with dementia and their carers want and need, or accept what help we have.

If you have no family and no money, staying home is hard. You'll need help—but Medicaid won't send you an aide unless you or a competent family member or even a neighbor will accept responsibility for supervising the helper. Even when there is a family, the job of caregiving is so much harder than anything that most hardworking people have ever done. We need and have only begun to build a network of support, in which the person with dementia can depend on family and/or paid caregivers, and those caregivers can depend in turn on others. The caregivers need help, too—a lot more than most get now. They need education about the illness; they need training in how to do specific things that a person with dementia might need; they need respite; they need to know that they will also be cared for when their time comes. Without all this in place, we will not be able to help people with dementia—and that's millions of people—stay home as they would like. Money makes a difference, of course, but it's not the only ingredient needed for success, and not always the most important one. Mrs. T had a meaningful experience caring for a demented spouse at home, though it wasn't easy. Mrs. S had a harder time, though she devoted herself to seeing that her husband had good care. Mrs. D, with her pigeons, was alone and in danger. She didn't want or accept any help. There was no way to do what she wanted and keep her and her neighbors safe. We ignore caregivers at our peril. They are the safety net. They are the key to living with dementia.

Chapter 11

Try a Little Tenderness

Here is a way to whistle in the dark, to help you imagine a dementia that contains joy. The capacity to enjoy and respond to music outlasts many other cognitive functions; even after spontaneous speech has become difficult, many people can still sing lyrics to songs learned long ago. Even in advanced disease, when happiness is hard to come by, people can respond to music they love. So I've borrowed a good idea; I'm going to go ahead and make my playlist now, to help me picture being happy, even with dementia.[1] I haven't dressed it up to impress you. (As Louis Jordan would say, "Makes no difference what you think about me; makes a whole lotta difference what I think about you.") This is mostly the music of my youth. I danced with heedless abandon to some of these songs; some call up images of those I love. This is the music with the best chance to wake me, if only for a moment, when I have fully entered the realm of tiny Hibernian warrior princesses.

"Let's Groove," Earth, Wind & Fire
"Respect," Aretha Franklin (or "Ain't No Way"; I'm torn,
    but we're going nowhere without Aretha)

"Beans and Cornbread," Louis Jordan

"Move On Up," Curtis Mayfield

"Get Down On It," Kool & the Gang

"Let's Stay Together," Al Green

"I'll Take You There," The Staple Singers

"St. Thomas," Sonny Rollins (my husband's favorite)

"For What It's Worth," Buffalo Springfield (older child
performed this in high school with my husband)

"Compared to What," Ray Charles

"Brick House," The Commodores

"Always Be My Baby," Mariah Carey (both children)

"You Can Close Your Eyes," James Taylor (my younger
daughter, her lullaby)

"Like a Rolling Stone," Bob Dylan

"Try a Little Tenderness," Otis Redding Jr.

"I'll Be Seeing You," Billie Holliday

This playlist helps me create a positive image of living with dementia, which I find hard to do. Your playlist will be different, but you should try making one. They help you look back over your life, collect a few moments of joy—or even sorrow—to bring forward to the future, for a time when it won't be easy for you to look back. It will be your gift to yourself with dementia. A small gift, I admit, in the face of a big problem. But what I hope, for both you and me, is to shift our view. Dementia is not all horror all the time. Try a little tenderness toward your future self.

Dementia is frightening, no doubt about it. Somewhere between a third and a half of Americans will have it by the time they reach eighty-five.[2] I assume I'm in the batch that has it, and a lot of you will be in that group, too. I don't like it, but there you have it. Our identities are tied up with our ability to remember—to conjure up our mother's smile, the scent of the baby's head after her bath. We take pride in our ability to do well the things we have learned to do. The loss of those hard-won abilities is tough; we feel it keenly even before it happens. That fear prevents us from facing the future, and that failure will mean our lives with dementia will not be as full and as happy as they might be.

Dementia's onset is slow; the day of diagnosis is not the day of oblivion. You can choose to see that gradual loss as a glass half empty or half full. The half-empty version is easier to see. That's why we should consider the half-full version. Many of us will live with the reality of dementia, of losing our cognitive abilities bit by bit. Are there ways to find joy? Adapting an adage borrowed from hospice, how can we make every remaining day a good day?

Some readers may balk at the idea of finding any pleasure within dementia. They see themselves bed-bound, incontinent, drooling. They don't want their family to ever see them that way. I ask you to bear with me. I am talking here about the beginning of dementia, not the end. Most people with the disease are walking about, joining the family at birthdays and summer picnics. Mild to moderate dementia lasts for years—so it was for my mother and grandmother. During that phase, a person enjoys many of the things she always enjoyed, like the company of family and friends. Some activities are no longer possible, but many remain not only feasible but enjoyable. I don't mean to whitewash the reality of living with the disease. But if there is a way to survive or maybe even thrive with dementia, I'd like to know about it.

Living a good life with dementia means maintaining independence and dignity, as much and as long as possible, in the presence of cognitive disability. Paradoxically, accepting help is the best way to maintain independence. But what help, when? We will be vulnerable, but what protections, if any, make sense? It is hard to get the balance right. Most people with mild to moderate symptoms live at home. They need, either on their own or with help, to keep a clean enough and safe enough home, get their meals, see friends and family, do things they enjoy, and get to the doctor, to their place of worship, and to wherever else they need to go.

I am not ignoring dementia's end stage. I am saying that fear of the ending prevents us from taking steps to improve life earlier on. That fear is not just about dementia, but about something more slippery, something psychological. We loathe the picture of ourselves as weakened, as frail and impaired. Perhaps you see yourself as a doer, a decider. That image, of course, is not the whole truth. You depend on other people. Dependence, even weakness, is part of the human condition. You were incontinent at birth, and you may be again before you die. I don't minimize the inconvenience of incontinence or other disabling physical problems. But practical issues can be addressed; what upsets us more is the symbolic weight of returning to an infant's helplessness. That's a problem of perspective and can be looked at in more than one way. For example, disabled people frequently rate the quality of their lives higher than clinicians and the general public do.[3] Living with a challenge, physical or cognitive, is consistent with a good life. Disabled people prove this every day. Our own growing disability is an unavoidable part of aging. We need to figure out how to find happiness within that reality, or we will not be happy. There is no other option.

I am not a natural optimist. I don't feel cheerful about tackling this challenge. Just the opposite. I am very attached to my brain. Truthfully, I am a terrible intellectual snob. As an academic I attend a lot of conferences, and I've heard some inspiring, insightful talks. But I'd be embarrassed if you knew how often I sat in the audience thinking,

"Who has let this braying donkey get up onstage?" I am a lifelong bookworm. I am a medical school professor. I love teaching subtle and complex concepts, trying to pique the interest of a future generation. I went to school forever and was absurdly competitive there. I loved that. It is a crushing blow to think of myself growing less sharp by the day. But I see the need to forge a way forward with a changing self and a changing brain. I may not succeed. Ironically, I would feel stupid for not trying, and that I cannot tolerate.

Here is the great lesson of optimism: If you let a problem overwhelm you, you won't look for and won't find solutions. If you at least look, you may discover some ways to engineer improvements. You don't actually have to feel optimistic. You just have to act as if a solution is possible. To tackle a problem, you break it down, looking for bugs you might successfully beat; you try partial solutions, see what works, and knit the fixes together as best you can. In tackling dementia, the overall solution of a cure will not arrive in time for me or the rest of the baby boomers. But we can improve our quality of life for years by diminishing specific obstacles.

I'm going to look at a handful of dementia's challenges and see how to get closer to the goal of a happy demented life. I'll consider activities I might enjoy with dementia. I'll look at symptoms most likely to cause trouble. Memory loss is what people associate with dementia, but that's not exactly what makes it hard for you to stay happy or stay home. Wandering, agitation, and incontinence are all more troublesome. Big problems also come with driving, sex, and money. These are trouble spots; that's where we'll need help. I don't know if these fixes will work or for how long. I am trying to rescue my future by constructing a picture where joy is still possible. Just trying to do this has helped me feel better today, because I'm less afraid. If it helps me enjoy tomorrow, that will be a bonus.

I'm going to plan for late onset dementia, as my mother and grand-mother had, and which millions of us will develop. Of course, I hope to delay its onset through exercise, diet, and cognitive engagement. But let's say my virtuous efforts fail, and I develop dementia in my seventies, just as my mother did. What will help me extend my time, not just of living but of happiness?

I'll be at home then, most likely. I hope my husband will be home with me. He's a good bet for healthy aging, with his whippet-thin frame and admirable habits. But virtue does not guarantee a long life together. So I hope I'll be part of a team, but I can't know that for sure. If I am, that will help me stay home longer.

I hate having nothing to do—and my demented mother hated that, too. Keeping me busy will be good for me and whoever cares for me. Finding activities compatible with dementia is my first design prob-lem. Embarrassment about forgetting names or the rules of the weekly card game can lead people to withdraw, increasing the likelihood of depression and more loss of function. Today there are many programs out there for people with mild to moderate symptoms. I'll need to find out what I can do, including new ways to be out and about with oth-ers. I've never been big on groups, but I'm looking to change my atti-tude. Most dementia support groups require a caregiver and offer a chance to socialize and escape the boredom and isolation of home. You can try a museum program; some are based on the popular Meet Me at MoMA.[4] If your community doesn't have a program that fits you, volunteering now to set one up would help others and your future self.

I hope I can garden through the early stages—I have loved garden-ing since childhood, when my mother let me plant a rose garden in a corner of our backyard. My favorite birthday present for several years was the chance to choose a new rosebush. I spent hours poring over glossy catalogues, agonizing over which one to pick. Sadly, I learned that these pinup shots may not resemble the scraggly thing in your garden; that's how gardeners grow. I have a garden now, and there are community gardens nearby. It doesn't matter if I can name the plants or if I can do much digging. It makes me happy to sit and look at plants, to see which the birds and butterflies visit. I will build that into my plan. Community gardens that promote multigenerational participation provide social connection, so that's an added benefit. Gardening moves inside during northern winters. A forgetful gardener can easily kill plants with kindness, overwatering them until they drown. It's much harder to kill a plant by misting it, though, so you could let a demented gardener mist plants all day, keeping her cheerful through the colder months.

Reading is another problem I need to tackle. As a little girl, I used to hide in quiet places to read, away from my five brothers and sisters. We had a three-story-tall pine tree in front of our house that I used to climb way up until I reached a hidden spot, where I read for hours. I no longer read in trees, but I haven't really changed. Reading is my solace and my celebration. It is my addiction. I ride the New York subway to work instead of driving so I can read. Some of the people I most admire and whose company I most enjoy are fictional characters. It makes me sad to think that as dementia rolls in, brain fog will limit my reading.

But maybe I can adapt. Kay Redfield Jamison, in *An Unquiet Mind*, her lovely memoir of coping with bipolar illness, took up children's books when illness made reading difficult.[5] If *Wind in the Willows* is good enough for Jamison, it's good enough for me. I'll stick with good books, but different ones. I read to my children when they were young, as my mother did for me. We have those books at home, and my family can point me toward them. An added bonus: A weak memory is a benefit, not a liability, when you read favorites over and over. You don't have to recall what you read yesterday; you can just read the same book again, with the same happy result. I see no loss of dignity in delighting in a book, regardless of its intended audience. I happily anticipate return visits to Stuart Little, Madeline, *Bartholomew and the Oobleck*, and *No Fighting, No Biting!* When I can't read, I might enjoy listening to a children's book on tape; I'll add these to my playlist. After a time, I'll have to give up books—I realize that. But I'd like to see how adaptation can extend my time doing what I love. Reading won't fix the larger problem of having dementia, but it might make me happy for a while. That's a start.

I anticipate carping from those who think it wrong to point older people with dementia toward children's activities. Indeed, there is a lively debate about whether it's infantilizing and wrong for demented people to play with doll babies, which some enjoy.[6] My view: If a thing makes my demented self happy and hurts no one else, I should do that thing. Moreover, playing with a doll may mean I don't have to use something worse to calm my agitation. For the last several years there has been a major push to decrease the inappropriate use of antipsychotic medications in nursing homes. These drugs have serious side effects (delirium, hospitalization, hip fracture, mortality) and are not especially effective at treating agitation, for which they are commonly used.[7] Aside from being risky and ineffective, they can also be extremely expensive. Calming an agitated person with a dolly is by no means the worst option.

In addition to dolls, there is a robot baby seal named Paro, with great big eyes, which is used to calm demented patients, effectively substituting for medications; these toys serve a serious purpose. Some object to Paro, either because it "tricks" impaired people into thinking it's real or because we should always use humans instead of robots for care.[8] I find neither of those arguments persuasive. My goal is to safely comfort those with cognitive impairment, and if fake pets work, bring them on. My only objection to Paro is his $6,000 price tag. Hasbro has since come up with a $95 kitty called Joy for All Tabby Cat, with a picture of a confused grandma on the box cover.[9] Fewer bells and whistles, same idea. They both purr; neither one scratches. (I would love to see a head-to-head comparative effectiveness study of the two.) We don't have enough human carers to go around, and the ratio of workers to needy people is falling. When we don't have enough people, we've fallen back on restraints, first physical and more recently chemical. I'd rather have the safer, cheaper, cuter robo-kitty.

As I mentioned, music offers an important path toward joy for those with cognitive impairments. The playlist that opens this chapter is based on the work of the Music & Memory program, which trains workers to create individualized play lists on iPods for nursing home residents, based on their positive responses.[10] A wonderful documentary shows a severely demented and withdrawn patient begin to smile, hum, and tap his feet when his nurse presses play.[11] You can't help wanting to join him. You may have read about or met someone with dementia who can still sing and play music. That takes us back to the Unforgettables, the chorus we met at the start of this book, in which carers and people with dementia sing together, sweeping up listeners in the tide of joy.

Music has so many benefits in dementia that it pops up all over the world. The UK Alzheimer's Society sponsors Singing for the Brain, popular weekly singing groups for those with dementia, incorporating playful exercises and games.[12] The U.S. Alzheimer's Association devotes a page to music therapy, and quotes Oliver Sacks: "Music evokes emotion, and emotion can bring with it memory."[13] I am not much of a singer, but I do love to dance, which helps slow cognitive decline.[14] The National Ballet School of Canada and the Baycrest Centre for

Geriatric Care are developing an evidence-based dance therapy program specifically for those with dementia.[15] I hope I'll still have a way to enjoy music if I develop dementia, through singing, dancing, or just listening. Enjoying music in a group is also a companionable activity that precludes conversation, perfect for the word-challenged person.

I love walking, but that can be either a liability or an asset here. Exercise generally slows cognitive decline and improves mood, and walking gets you out of the house. But people with dementia get lost, and they can get into real trouble. Twenty-five years ago, when there was less awareness of this problem, an older man with dementia failed to return to his apartment in New York City; his adult daughter called the police. They didn't see the need to search for him—he had no obligation to tell his daughter where he was. His body was found days later near the Hudson River. That incident inspired a push to protect lost dementia patients. Jed Levine, executive vice president of CaringKind, formerly the New York City branch of the Alzheimer's Association, notes that in New York City, nearly one person with dementia gets lost each day.[16] CaringKind and the NYPD sponsor a registry system that records name and contact information on a wristband. There are also phone apps that let you track other people, as long as they keep their phone with them. Technological solutions are getting better and more numerous, but wandering remains a major reason for someone's no longer being safe at home.

In 2010, the UK sponsored a design contest to create solutions for dementia's challenges, and some clever Scottish students tackled the problem of wandering by training service dogs for people with dementia.[17] The dog would leave the house with the person. Dog and human would be out and about, chatting with neighbors and letting local kids pat the dog. The dog decreases isolation and increases exercise—two good ways to promote both happiness and health. The dog knows the way home and gets his person safely there. Dementia dogs can be trained to help their people remember to eat, drink, and take medications. One pooch licks his owner's arm where a medication patch should go, as a helpful reminder. A dog doesn't solve all problems, of course. It is still risky to head outside in the dead of night or in the bitter cold. Dogs can be time-consuming and expensive to train. The UK Dementia Dog Project solves this problem through innovative programs, like a course that gives prisoners job skills by teaching them to train service dogs;[18] their pups are more affordable than many. Most important, though, a dog can buy time at home. Such a simple, low-tech, tail-wagging solution. Good dog!

Gardening, reading, walking—these don't constitute a detailed guide for living with dementia, not for you and not even for me. They are first steps on the path toward seeing myself as a happy person, with dementia. They are a way to push back against the fear-mongering image of dementia as the bitterest of endings. I hope they will permit me to tackle additional serious challenges, instead of avoiding the whole mess altogether. A life with dementia for you will look different. But if you don't create the image you'd like to see, someone else will design your life, and it may not suit you half as well.

As my dementia progresses, I will need more care. What should that look like? Starting about twenty years ago, scholars worked hard to redefine how we see the person with dementia, in part to help reexamine what sort of care such a person needs. In *The Moral Challenge of Alzheimer's Disease,* for example, Stephen Post argues that our society places too great a premium on cognition, and that this is not the cardinal feature of a person.[19] The capacity to feel emotions, to experience well-being or its absence, to respond to kindness and cruelty, all remain for the person with dementia, and are a better basis for respect than cognitive function. For Post, people with dementia should not be viewed as the sum of their losses, but rather as people with assets and liabilities, more like than unlike others. Building on a person's remaining strengths enhances function and quality of life. Post's work influenced important changes in dementia care, ranging from the overall culture of nursing homes to a stronger emphasis on quality of life.

The late Tom Kitwood was admired—revered, really—for his work on affirming the humanity of people with dementia. He specifically attacked the link between no cure and no care. His seminal book, *Dementia Reconsidered: The Person Comes First*, opens with a story about an advocacy group that requested photos of his patients to use for fundraising.[20] Dutifully, the staff sent photos of the cheerful residents. The photos were rejected. Those pictured were nowhere near "disturbed and agonized" enough for the promotional campaign. The advocacy group hoped to portray the horrors of dementia, as so many do. Kitwood worked toward just the opposite goal. He rejected the idea that an incurable disease presents a grim future for patient and carer. He saw benefits for both givers and receivers of good dementia care. In Kitwood's view, caring for those with dementia can "take us out of our customary patterns of over-busyness, hypercognitivism and extreme talkativity, into a way of being in which emotion and feeling are given a much larger place."[21] Kitwood stressed the enduring value, the personhood, of those with dementia. Rather than demonize them with photos of agony, he emphasized recognition, respect, and trust. Authors like Kitwood and Post paint a portrait of a whole person. Long ago, British physician Thomas Wakley called the workhouse the antechamber of the grave. Today, thoughtful experts work to create dementia care that does not just kill time until death, but offers a way to live well.

I find in this philosophy of dementia care a form of modern moral treatment, though not labeled as such by its practitioners. The emphasis on the dignity of the person with dementia echoes the nineteenth century's radical approach to people with mental illness, promoting compassion and removing punishment. The new version of moral treatment does not suggest that kindness will cure dementia. It combines compassion with contemporary neuroscience. It acknowledges damage to specific types of cognitive function and relies on remaining skills to foster communication and reduce symptoms like agitation and anxiety. As with the original nineteenth-century approach, many of these new programs rely on design of the physical environment, communication styles, and activity programs, more than on pharmacological methods.

Take, for instance, the work of John Zeisel, a design expert who was once asked to fix problems at an assisted living facility. That modest request radically altered the course of his professional life, leading him to become an expert in promoting wellness for those with dementia.[22] Like Thomas Kirkbride, an early proponent of moral treatment, Zeisel was horrified to find patients tied to their beds and chairs. Zeisel saw the problem of the wandering demented person as a design challenge, one that must have a better solution than lashing a person miserably in place. Why not create spaces for people with dementia that permit free movement while maintaining safety? He disguised the exits of dementia units to reduce the risk of a person leaving unobserved. He designed circular walking routes and multiple cues to help residents stay oriented and avoid panic. He kept floors clear of rugs and clutter to minimize falls. In the past, people institutionalized with dementia were often kept indoors for years on end. Influenced by Zeisel and others, many facilities now include fenced gardens and other safe, pleasant outdoor spaces that residents can visit at liberty.

Zeisel, working with psychologist Paul Raia, argued that though dementia has no cure, that need not mean no treatment.[23] They didn't choose kindness or science; they chose both. They looked at how dementia changes the way a person "thinks, feels, communicates."[24] They expanded their focus beyond memory loss and looked at the preservation of emotional connection and the loss of language skills and impulse control. They used this knowledge to design programs that preserve function and work around deficits, calling their approach *habilitation*. This approach does not attempt to restore lost function, as in re-habilitation, but works with function still retained. Their main goal is simple: "Bring about a positive emotion and maintain [it] for as long as possible."[25] They want people with dementia to feel happy. Sounds good to me. And in addition, their approach also slows the progression of the disease and decreases the use of medication.

Habilitation and similar approaches teach workers to communicate effectively with people with dementia. Words alone don't change a problematic behavior in someone whose language skills are fading; the simple repetition of a verbal instruction is useless. In this approach, workers are taught to change their own behavior or the environment. (This is an adaptable piece of wisdom. An old friend of mine is a rower whose coach told the team, "When you are sure that someone else in the boat is creating a problem, change what you are doing." This rights the rocking boat every time.) Addressing the cause of the behavior is a better way to change it than telling a nonverbal person to stop. If agitation is caused by pain, treat the pain. If aggression is caused by fear, remove what is scary.

Habilitation does not wrench the person with dementia into our world, but invites caregivers to meet the person in theirs (like that midnight train to Georgia). Distraction is acceptable; a weaponized truth is not. This technique can be used in the classic problem of a man who doesn't recall his wife has died. Caregivers do not conceal the truth, but neither do they force him to grieve every day by repeating the news. A skilled caregiver, when asked by this man where his (dead) wife is, will turn the question to one side rather than confront it head on. They might say, "I guess she's not here right now. But I know you have photos of her in your scrapbook. Let's look at them while we wait, and you can tell me about her."

Now we have to tackle a really touchy issue: incontinence. There, I've said it. Both potential patients and caregivers regard it with horror. But even *it* doesn't have to stop joy in its tracks. We have another engineering problem: How do we manage leaking body fluids without mess, embarrassment, or undue restriction? It's not a new question. Babies have this problem, and frankly, so does every woman who has menstruated. You can't have a city if you don't deal with sewage, and you can't have a happy person if you don't deal with hers. A good nursing home helps dementia patients use the toilet regularly, especially after meals. Better, smaller, drier adult diapers would help, ones that are not embarrassing or uncomfortable to wear—maybe ones that look like underwear (tighty-whities, not boxers). Where there is a market, there will be innovation and improvement. In Japan, more adult diapers are now sold than infant ones. Incontinence is a serious challenge, not a moral failing or a reason to kill yourself. It is a design problem, one that I hope smart people will take on.

Effective dementia care solves problems that trouble the patient, not just the helpers. But tackling these problems helps caregivers, too. Everyone wins. Finding solutions for a person who wanders, stays awake all night, or cries out in agitation means that this person can live more peacefully with whoever is near them. If that's your family, you'll be able to stay home longer. If those are your companions in the nursing home, you will feel better and be treated better, and won't be asked to leave. This care is different from warehousing patients as they wait for death. This care is possible today. It does not require the presence of angels or unaffordable staffing levels. It requires sustained leadership and a commitment to adequate training. It requires an approach to the individual person with dementia that looks to make her happy and comfortable. When I get there, that's what I want.

There is one other activity I'll mention. I volunteer for dementia-related research, and I hope to continue this in the years to come. I feel strongly that bioethicists should volunteer for medical research. We talk a good game about how important it is to protect and inform participants, and about why other people, specifically minorities, should volunteer. It's time for us to step up. The need for volunteers is nowhere more urgent than in the domain of dementia. NIH estimates that 70,000 volunteers will be needed in the next decade or so, and that recruiting research subjects is among the biggest obstacles to making progress.[26] I stalled for a while before participating in research. I have many excuses. I am busy. I am a physical coward. But now I have signed up. Scientists will learn more about dementia if they can do more research, and that research may benefit me or my family.

Before jumping in, I decided to investigate what it would take to get involved, and modeled my efforts on Nancy Drew. She first appeared back in 1930 as an attractive sixteen-year-old blonde, setting out for her adventures in a blue roadster. Today she would be well over a hundred. If she's going to investigate dementia, she'll need a suitable assistant. How about a silver-haired medical school professor, one who usually sets out for her adventures via the urinous 125th Street station of New York City's 4 train? Nancy often got into scrapes in her work, like getting locked in the closet of an abandoned cabin. It seems fair that her assistant—that would be me—should also put her body on the line. So that's what I'll do.

First, I needed a study that would accept me, which was trickier than I'd anticipated. I'm not old enough for studies focused on the elderly and I don't have dementia, though I do have a family history. On the plus side, I am a doctor, so I'm not scared of most medical tests. I am willing (mostly) to fill out endless forms about my medical or family history. I do have my limits, however. I am not willing to take an experimental medicine that is not yet FDA approved for a condition I don't have (dementia) in the hopes of preventing it. But someone else might.

Searching on the web, I found the Brain Health Registry, run by researchers at UCSF.[27] It looked like fun! You play brain games. You fill out questionnaires about your sleep, diet, mood, and health history. They'll check back in with you every three to six months and ask you to repeat the games, to see how your noggin is coming along. They hope to collect a huge data set to help figure out which changes in cognitive function predict the development of dementia.

I found their site while I was on the train home from Washington, DC. I cheerfully filled out lots of demographic data. Easy! The website encouraged me to find a quiet place to take the cognitive tests. The train was not optimal, but I often work well in noisy places, so I forged ahead. Did the lurching train, spotty internet, and overhead announcements make a difference? Who knows, but I did poorly. I had to push a button if a card I'd seen before popped up on my screen, but I didn't know if the test batch of cards counted as "seen before." I got one wrong. I panicked. I didn't know how to pause and collect myself. The cards kept coming and I got a whole batch wrong in a row. My upper lip was sweating. I was light-headed. A great weight of sorrow descended upon me. I saw cognitive impairment coming right at me, not in theory, but in reality and right now. I turned my face to the window and saw a grim self-portrait in the ruined warehouses, their windows gouged out. I placed a hand quietly on my husband's comforting arm while he read. I decided to take no more tests on the train.

The next morning, feeling low, I kept picturing my mother in the throes of dementia. In her youth, she had been fiercely competitive, skipping grades, always striving. She held us to high academic standards by simply assuming we would meet them. (Six kids, six graduate degrees.) She was nearly unbeatable at Boggle. But I recalled a day late in her life when she was in the nursing home, failing at Parcheesi, a kindhearted attendant coaching her as she moved her wizened little player around the board.

My first low-risk experience as a research participant was far harder than I expected. You don't have to be a board-certified psychiatrist to draw a few conclusions here, but as it happens, I am one. I have seen dementia up close and don't want to go there. I also know I might. I hadn't realized it ahead of time, but I was terrified of these innocent-seeming tests. A few wrong answers might prove not only that I was doomed to develop dementia someday but also that today was the day. Contemplating the reality of cognitive decline ripped a large hole in my safety net. I felt the sense of joy and expectation about the months and years ahead break apart, like an iceberg sliding into the sea. I jumped into the task of participating in research as an intellectual exercise, a kind of game, but stumbled across more serious psychological territory than I expected.

After a breather, I pulled myself together and discovered another website, this one for the MindCrowd study,[28] which is trying to get a million people to sign up and take cognitive tests so they too can amass data to study what goes into losing or maintaining mental function. Ready to take my lumps, I sat before the screen and was presented with a batch of word pairs. The screen then displayed one word in the pair and asked me to type in its companion word. This I could do. No nervous feeling, no distractions. This small success helped heal my wounded pride.

I persevered and found that New York University was looking for healthy volunteers in my age range, so off I went on the odiferous 4 train, Nancy Drew style, to see what they were up to. I had to skip food and drink from the night before my visit and couldn't have coffee until after some blood tests. That bothered me a great deal. I am sullen and simpleminded without that one cup of morning coffee.

At NYU, I met Rachel (not her real name) in the soaring lobby. She was a charming foot soldier in the vast army of young people who work for a year or two after college, apprenticing themselves to huge research institutions while applying to medical school. Rachel escorted me to the blood-testing lab and gave me lengthy and repetitive forms to fill out. As I worked away, another coordinator sat beside me, accompanied by another participant, a frail woman in her late seventies who had trouble filling out the forms. She asked a few anxious questions and received reassurance, as much from the comforting tone of the coordinator as by her answers. She signed a form saying she understood the research was unlikely to benefit her directly. Many people sign such forms and still hope they will be the one who gets lucky, benefiting from the newest, best treatment for what ails them.

I then sat in a crowded waiting room until a man called my name, took down the same information I'd already given, and sent me off to donate several vials of blood and some pee in the familiar cup. After the lab, I was given $10 to get breakfast. I sprinted to the kiosk across the hall. Huge coffee, modest muffin: At the right moment, these are things that make life worth living. I bolted the coffee, afraid that further delay would mean a nasty headache. With burned tongue but clear mind, I took up my research duties again.

Next stop: a clinical research center at NYU, now called the Center for Cognitive Neurology, where I met a physician I will call Dr. X. She was cordial and correct. Her job was to give me a physical exam and ask about my medical history. Dr. X was skeptical that I wanted to volunteer just to help other people. She was right, of course; my participation was in fact a form of research. I felt a bit sneaky. She had to get approval for her research and tell me about any risks. As a participant, I didn't have those same obligations. No regulation prevents me from writing about my experience or requires me to inform the researcher. I did participate fully, answering all questions accurately and not concealing my identity. Still, I wasn't sharing something, and she smelled a rat. Dr. X kept asking questions about my concerns regarding dementia. I said I was there to help others, and that bioethicists should participate in research—a true but incomplete answer. She appeared to want me to say that my function was in decline, which had prompted my enrollment. There are studies showing that those who complain about memory changes are good at predicting their own decline. But that is not my situation. I *am* worried about dementia but in the long run. I am at risk, as are many of us, but I don't have it today. To be sure, my memory is not what it was when I was twenty; modest changes are typical for someone in middle age. Reaction times slow normally; concentration wanes. I don't remember names and retrieve other sorts of information as quickly as I used to, and I'll give you a dollar if you can find someone older than fifty who can.

Still, Dr. X was suspicious. She asked if I made more lists than previously to keep track of tasks. I answered yes and she wrote this down. I pointed out that I have more responsibilities and staff than I used to. She gave me a tolerant smile, but did not write *that* down. She asked me what was the major news event of the day before and I had no idea. (The Senate had released a controversial report on CIA interrogation.) It had been a jam-packed day; I got home late after a work-related dinner. Even then I had to sign some documents to go in the mail the next morning. The day of my interview with Dr. X began with a meeting at home with a contractor about a home renovation. I had rushed to NYU and answered work email on the train. I usually read the paper every morning but had not done so that day. I paused, knowing that lengthy explanations create an impression of guilt. I told Dr. X I'd had a busy twenty-four hours and had never known yesterday's big event to begin with, so I had not had the opportunity to forget it. She wrote that down, too. This time I was better prepared for the effect of being under the magnifying lens and suffered no psychological distress. I proceeded to the next cog in the research machine.

This cog was Seamus (not his real name either), a cheery red-bearded youngster, so Irish he might have been dressed all in green with a pointy hat. I couldn't help picturing him as an altar boy. Seamus was to administer my cognitive tests. Off we went to a windowless room with two chairs, a desk, and a computer. Like the Catholic Stations of the Cross, we progressed through an aptly named battery of tests. He told me three things to remember and asked me to repeat them back again after a few minutes. He showed me a geometric figure and asked me to draw it from memory. He read me some paragraphs and I repeated them back with as many tedious details as possible. He read me strings of numbers; each time I repeated a string correctly, he would dial up the challenge and present me with another longer one. Next, he recited more number strings but asked me to repeat them backward, a loathsome activity that made my brain tired. At length we came to my favorite, word pairs, which I rocked, just as I had done for the MindCrowd study. I know vocabulary is generally preserved with aging, but one celebrates the victories one can. On and on we went, until at last Seamus released me from my penance.

Seamus was warm and encouraging and managed to make me feel competent, whether I answered all questions correctly or not. As Dickens observed in *David Copperfield*, a supportive teacher helps a person perform better; I left feeling as if I still had a few more good years after all. I was surprised to find how different this experience was from taking those first tests for the computer registry. Perhaps a broader range of tests reminded me I am more capable in some domains than others—true of every human on the planet. In any case, having the right person as a guide makes a big difference. I recall sitting with my mother once while a physician peppered her with questions: Who is the president? Who ran in the last election? He was cold and lacking in empathy. My mother could not answer and was enraged at the doctor, at herself, at the whole stinking mess of memory loss. She did not have much memory, but she knew when she'd been humiliated.

I participated in a study investigating the links between sleep, oxygen, and cognition. It required me to don some kinky sleep paraphernalia. Velcro straps! Now we're having fun! One strap went across my chest, another across my belly; the buttons in between looked as if they might blow me up. A clear plastic tube looped around each ear and plugged into my nose. I was to sleep this way for three nights while the device recorded my activity levels and oxygen use. On the morning of the fourth day I anticipated waking from my slumbers, not like a princess, but like a woman with a seriously irritated spouse.

I had a brain MRI. I put all my clothes, including anything metal, into a locker. (MRIs work through magnets and can yank metal things, including heavy oxygen tanks, across the room.) In the machine, a woven plastic basket was placed over my face, like a tomato basket from the grocery store but in the shape of a fencing mask. I lay on a stretcher and was rolled back into a sort of coffin lit like a shopping mall. I closed my eyes and tried to fall asleep, while still remembering not to move even the least bit. Then *bang bang bang!* There followed a series of trumpet blasts and loud hums, like really terrible atonal music. I would hear a different note on the horn and then more loud hums. It was mildly irksome, but otherwise okay. There is no radiation involved, unlike with a CT scan, and MRIs cause no known harm unless you have metal ensconced in your body. (Cyborgs beware.)

I participate in research to help increase knowledge about dementia. Maybe this will help others one day. It is not going to help me, at least not directly. I won't learn the results of any of my tests (unless maybe they find something major like a tumor that requires vigorous action on my part). I would like to learn what it means to be a research subject and ask how we might make that experience better. It is difficult to get people to enroll in research, and unless they do, we won't learn as much and as quickly as we could.

But why don't more people volunteer? There is the potential threat to one's sense of well-being, but the problem is bigger than that. People are afraid. They don't trust researchers to tell them the truth, to protect them from injury, and to treat them with respect. These beliefs can't be dismissed out of hand—there have been some horrific scandals in which participants were greatly harmed. The most famous was the long-running Tuskegee study of syphilis, funded by the U.S. Public Health Service, in which African American men were deliberately not told they had syphilis and thus were prevented from getting treatment so that doctors could learn how untreated syphilis affects the body. Guess what they found, after forty years? Syphilis is bad for you. Though the study was never secret, it went unnoticed for decades. When it came to public attention in the 1970s, the disgrace helped build the modern structure of research regulation.

And there have been many others. A landmark *New England Journal* article from 1966 by Henry Beecher provided a catalogue of horrors, collected by the simple method of reviewing prestigious medical journals and pulling out ethically questionable studies.[29] (Though Beecher anonymized the papers he chose, they have since been identified by historian David Rothman.[30]) Beecher's examples are chilling. For me, the most upsetting was an intimate affair involving only one subject, published in 1965.[31] A woman was dying of melanoma. Her mother, hoping to help, permitted researchers to stitch a sample of her daughter's tumor to her own abdominal muscles. What they learned is that this is a good way to kill someone. The previously healthy mother died fifteen months later, after multiple grueling surgeries and long hospital stays, from melanoma. The authors offer no apology and express no sorrow. They note that "it was felt at the time that there was probably no risk." They never say, "We were wrong." This grieving mother was murdered as much as if she'd been shot by a gun to the head, all in the name of science.

The world of research today is a different and highly regulated one. Current oversight is not perfect but would prevent a study like Tuskegee or one that gives a mother her daughter's fatal cancer. We require that participants or an appropriate surrogate get full information, evaluate the risks and benefits, and give informed consent. At academic medical centers, pharmaceutical firms, or any place that hopes for FDA approval for a new drug or device, review boards spend countless hours evaluating any study with human subjects. Controversies about risky studies or poor informed consent still emerge, but the scope of problems is on a different scale from those of a few decades ago. There is now a substantial federal apparatus looking over the shoulder of researchers—and that's as it should be. There are professional associations that focus on protecting research subjects, including Public Responsibility in Medicine and Research (PRIM&R, pronounced *primer*). What we haven't done effectively is to persuade the public that participating in research now is a safe and meaningful thing to do. And it is not only the public we've failed to persuade. Many doctors don't refer their patients for research, and patients don't know how to find studies on their own. That is very much the point of the web-based data registries—they don't rely on a doctor knowing about your interest in dementia.

I learned something from being a subject rather than a doctor. I found out I am worried about getting dementia—no surprise there. The hardest part was dealing with my own fears, but the actual research was no worse than a minor nuisance and sometimes was actually fun. It is no small thing to contribute to our scientific knowledge base. For me, participating in research was a meaningful thing to do. I enjoy working, and like the idea of continuing to contribute even if I develop dementia.

If you choose to participate in research, the knowledge you help create may help you, though more likely it will help the next generation. You can set the level of risk where you like. It may be that signing up for a brain data registry is the right step—no blood tests, no waiting room. Or perhaps you would be willing to try an experimental medication that could slow down or prevent dementia. It's up to you. But if you're worried enough about dementia to read this book, you should check out options. You might help move the dial on what we know. You might also decide that living with dementia is compatible with being useful and happy.

A person with advancing dementia may need protection, particularly in the risk-prone domains of sex, driving, and money. How do we preserve freedom for those with dementia, without leaving them to stumble unaware into terrible risks? In the spring of 2014, Henry

Rayhons, a seventy-eight-year-old state legislator from Iowa, was arrested. For what crime was this churchgoing pillar of the community hauled in? He allegedly had sex with his wife, seventy-eight-year-old Donna Lou Rayhons. Wait, what?

In better days the Rayhons, both previously widowed, met while singing in a church choir.[32] By all reports they had a happy and affectionate relationship. Over time, Mrs. Rayhons developed dementia. She was admitted to a nursing home, due to the intervention of her two adult daughters from a prior marriage. That's odd; generally the spouse determines the right time for nursing home admission. A meeting was called to set a care plan for Mrs. Rayhon. The medical team limited trips out of the nursing home with her husband—odd again! Did they think visits with her husband were unsafe? A social worker at the facility, at the urging of the daughters, documented a physician's assessment that Mrs. Rayhon was not capable of consenting to sex. A short time later, one of the daughters petitioned for and obtained permission to serve as her mother's guardian—though generally a spouse serves as the default decision-maker. These various developments suggest that the daughters and the nursing home staff, rightly or wrongly, did not see Mr. Rayhons as the right person to protect his wife.

Soon after the meeting at the nursing home, Mrs. Rayhons was moved from a single to a double room. A roommate then reported sounds of sex emitting from behind the curtain around Mrs. Rayhons's bed while Mr. Rayhons was visiting. Mr. Rayhons was arrested. All agree that Mrs. Rayhons was always happy to see her husband. There was no suggestion that she resisted sex or objected to it. I know only what's in the newspapers, and that information suggests that preventing the act was exactly the goal. But why an arrest? Was there no less public, less punitive way of mediating this dispute, of respecting the private behavior of married adults while also protecting a potentially vulnerable person? And is there only one vulnerable person here? The steps taken by Mrs. Rayhons's daughters suggest they may have viewed him as impaired, and perhaps sexually disinhibited. By taking the very public and humiliating step of an arrest, this family created a situation in which their unhappy story was chewed up and spit out in an international media blitz. Surely there was a better way.

The trial resulted in exoneration for Mr. Rayhons. It also revealed that people have very conflicting feelings about sex and dementia. Many of us don't like to think that old people, either with or without dementia, have sex. We don't think they do have sex, or even that they should. At the risk of sounding too psychiatric, I note that many people don't like to think of their parents having sex, an activity that was a necessary prerequisite to their existence.

But the problem is even broader. There are prejudicial ideas about people with any sort of disability engaging in sex. The fact that we don't acknowledge sexuality in differently abled people means that we provide poor medical care related to sexual feelings and behaviors and have no relevant policies, or stupid ones. We react in a panic. We end up arresting married people for having sex with their spouse.

At the heart of the debate is the central question of bioethics: How do we balance freedom and safety? (In bioethics terms, autonomy and beneficence.) The question of sexual relationships is just one of many that force us to reexamine priorities in caring for those with dementia. In *Being Mortal*, Atul Gawande asks us to look at the balance of safety versus independence that is forced upon aging people.[33] The same challenge faces us with the question of when an older person with cognitive impairments has the capacity to consent to sex.

So how should we address the issue of sex for older people, those with cognitive impairments, and those in nursing homes? Those are three separate questions, each with its own complications. First, let's examine the assumption that older people no longer have sexual behavior or feelings. This is simply untrue for many. Sexual behavior varies as much among older people as it does in the young; some remain sexually active into their eighties and nineties, though the percentage declines with age. Age does bring illnesses that interfere with sexual activities. Older men experience difficulties sustaining erections. Older women experience discomfort during intercourse as a result of menopausal changes. There are commonly available, though imperfect, methods to address both these problems. Prescription drugs for erectile dysfunction are blockbusters; the majority of adult American women have used a lubricant at least once while having sex.[34] In any case, aging does not eliminate the wish for intimacy, security, physical touch, and companionship—all reasons why people of any age engage in sexual behaviors. And there is nothing about aging that prevents loneliness. Even those who no longer engage in traditional sexual activities may still crave the comfortable presence of a sleeping companion.[35]

Cognitive impairment raises tough issues, not only of consent but of consequences. For elders, we can take pregnancy off the table, but all sexually active people, old or young, impaired or not, need support and education to promote safer options and regular screening to address sexually transmitted diseases.

Assessing a cognitively disabled person's capacity to consent to sex is complicated. There is no standard test that quickly and easily produces an airtight answer. The best approach relies on a careful, individualized assessment of decision-specific capacity. By that I mean that in order to evaluate whether you can freely consent to sex, it's not helpful to know if you can balance your checkbook. That's a different skill set. Your memory needs to be good enough to follow a conversation and express your values and preferences, but your score on a standard memory test is not especially relevant. A sensitive clinician needs to interview the people involved so they don't feel they are on trial. The impaired person's feelings toward a potential partner should be explored, along with the possibility of coercion or a quid pro quo.

All this assessing is most likely to happen in a nursing home. Adults who live at home don't usually face an inquisition when they have sex. (Though adult children do become rightly concerned about exploitative relationships.) Once you live in an institution, you lose a lot of privacy. Someone else is responsible for keeping you safe, and that includes during your sexual activities. The majority of nursing home residents have dementia. If that's you, you might not recall you are still married or may mistake another person for your spouse. A spouse or adult child may hate the idea of a sexual relationship blossoming in the nursing home. They may fear you are being exploited or acting against your own lifelong values. Alternatively, they may be glad you have discovered someone who makes you happy. Either way, a lot more people are in your business than if you lived at home.

You'd think nursing homes would all have effective plans for dealing with these issues; after all, sex is nothing new. They don't. Nursing homes are all over the map when it comes to sexuality. Some have long had thoughtful policies and staff trained to implement them. The Hebrew Home at Riverdale in New York posts its policy, first drafted in 1995 and regularly updated since, on its website.[36] This document describes the rights of residents to privacy and respect for sexual expression, and outlines a process for addressing who might need assessment of decision-making capacity for sexual behavior, who performs such an assessment, and what that assessment looks like. Many others have no policy and are squeamish about the whole idea. (This seems to have been the case for the facility where Donna Lou Rayhons lived.) In a statistically invalid experiment, I assigned my bioethics masters students to visit different local nursing homes and assisted living facilities, to get a sense of what life there might be like. Among the questions students could ask was whether there was a policy regarding sexual behavior. Answers varied remarkably. One place claimed with horror that the issue had never come up—an eyebrow-raising statement. Another took the opposite tack, immediately answering that older adults were not children and that this facility respected their rights and dignity. They permitted residents to room together if they wished and use the same bed; this applied to same-sex as well as heterosexual couples. This level of openness is unusual. Same-sex older couples have an even tougher time than straight ones in finding acceptance for sexual expression in nursing homes.

The Rayhons case did have one positive impact. The uproar made a lot more facilities think about how they handle sexual relationships among residents. More professionals read the relevant academic articles, including a thoughtful 2015 review by James Wilkins, arguing for a liberalized, individualized approach to sexual expression for nursing home patients.[37]

People with dementia have more traffic collisions than people who don't, between two and five times more.[38] Nonetheless, lots of people with dementia drive. People feel strongly about driving. It is convenient. In many places public transportation is slow, unpredictable, and uncomfortable. In suburbia and rural areas it may barely exist, and certainly not for the last mile that connects to a person's home. Driving also represents freedom, independence, and possibility. Americans like to think we could set off on a cross-country road trip just because we feel like it. Or we could just head to the Piggly Wiggly for ice cream, but either way, it feels like where we go and why is up to us when a car sits in our driveway. We hate to say goodbye to wheels that mean freedom.

If you have a relative with dementia, it's likely driving is, was, or will be a problem. How do you know when someone's driving is impaired? Should everyone with dementia just stop driving? Who can help you find out when driving is no longer safe, and how do you get someone to stop? These are all good questions, yet helpful answers are not as available as they should be. Mild dementia does not mean that someone's driving is necessarily a danger. On the other hand, dementia progresses to more serious impairment and greater risk.

Getting my own mother to stop driving didn't go smoothly. Though her vision and hearing were fine, she would get lost and panic. If roadwork created a detour, my mother had to leave the route she'd used for seventy-five years. She had no mental backup; once off her well-grooved path, she was utterly lost. I told my mother that as a doctor, I recommended she stop driving altogether before she put anyone else in danger. This just made her mad. My brother added that we would make sure she had someone to help her get around when she needed. She hated the sound of that. She was enraged, shaking her diminutive fist in my brother's face. That conversation inspired my brother to create my mother's best and last nickname: the THWP, or Tiny Hibernian Warrior Princess. We could have used more help in making this transition.

Since dementia is common, and driving problems are common within dementia, you'd think there would be lots of solutions. There are tools to address driving and dementia, but there is no commonly used and widely accepted method for assessing driving competence in dementia.[39] Many families ask their doctors to help assess and implement a good plan—and find that their doctor has no training or information on how to approach the problem. Even if the doctor knew what to do, it would be tough to incorporate a useful intervention into the ever fewer minutes of a medical appointment. For now, the best plan is to request referral to a specialist who assesses driving; some departments of motor vehicles do this or can recommend those who do. Big medical centers may have a department of rehabilitation that can provide assessment. Those experts find that people with dementia are more likely to drive off the road, drive too slowly, brake poorly, and make slow left turns.[40] One day—maybe one day soon—self-driving cars will help people with dementia get around safely and independently. While we're waiting, there are steps families can take. Some ask a physician to play bad cop and tell a family member with dementia not to drive, and that may work. Many families resort to subterfuge to stop a relative's driving. Keys may be "lost," a car may be "sent for repairs" or left disabled in the drive (for instance, by removing the battery) and never repaired. All of these tricks may work, but using them may trouble families.

These are solutions that create ethical challenges. When is it right to be, well, dishonest to protect someone with dementia? The issue comes up again and again regarding medication, leaving the family home, and any change that the family thinks is right but the person with dementia does not accept. Is it right to take advantage of dementia's symptoms in order to protect someone? The answer, ethically, is that it depends on both the motivation for the subterfuge and its impact. Start with candor. Explore whether your relative feels safe driving or is worried. Confide your own concerns and observations. If she agrees with you that it is better to stop, you don't need to be conniving, which can undermine the relationship you are trying to preserve. If your motives in stopping Grandma from driving are multiple, separate them out, as conflicts of interest can make your actions especially dodgy. Maybe Grandma's car would be a very nice extra vehicle for you or your teenage son. If your interests intrude, you are not really, or not only, thinking of what's best for her. Perhaps it would be best to sell the car and use the funds to help support her care. She might never know, but you would.

First, try honest approaches at communication. If they fail, consider subterfuge as one way to protect and promote the interests of the person with dementia. If it's the only way you can find, after diligent efforts, to preserve the dignity and protect the safety of your relative and those she might injure, then to me that lie is ethically justifiable. (Not everyone would agree. Specifically, Immanuel Kant, granddaddy of analytic philosophers, did not justify lying even to save a life. I would rather save the life and take the hit.) So those who leave the permanently disabled car in the driveway, when asked by their relative why he can't drive it, could say, "That car's no good anymore." This is a near-lie, meaning it is a true statement that doesn't express the full truth. You have kept Grandpa from running over someone's child, and you have not humiliated him by saying that he too is just no good anymore. No perfect solution exists here; we'll have to settle for the least bad option.

Though we honor independence, no one should drive who poses a danger to others. Finding the right solution for your family may be hard. If I still live in New York City and join the ranks of tiny Hibernian warrior princesses, it shouldn't be difficult for my family to stop my driving. Our public transportation could be more accessible, but it is better than in most stretches of America. And it is challenging to drive in New York City. I can still be independent without a car, but many others are not so lucky. Let's hope self-driving cars get here soon and are affordable. Meanwhile, you may have to work to figure out when and how to get those keys.

. . .

Losing the capacity to make your own decisions about sex and driving is bad enough. Losing the right to control your money is, for some, even more devastating. It is hard to overstate the scope of the problem. People over sixty-five make up 13 percent of the U.S. population, but control 34 percent of assets.[41] Financial capacity, defined as "the ability to independently manage one's financial affairs in a manner consistent with personal self-interest," can be one of the earliest deficits of cognitive function, even before a diagnosis of dementia.[42] Loss of financial judgment may mean that a lifetime's savings disappear just when they are needed for long-term care.

Controlling one's money is a symbolically important aspect of adulthood. It hurts to hand over that power to someone else—and is all the more difficult given that paranoia is a common symptom of dementia. But it turns out that the distrust elders feel is not misplaced. In one large sample, 4.7 percent of older people reported suffering financial exploitation. The annual amount of such abuse in the United States is estimated at $3 billion.[43] Sadly, most financial abuse is carried out by family members or others well known to the victim.[44] For couples in which one partner has dementia, the transition to the other's handling the finances can be painful, especially when this task has long been associated with being the man of the house.[45] All this adds up to a big headache, one that is better addressed early than late.

Clinicians are often asked for help with financial incapacity from distressed family members. As is true in the case of evaluations for sexual and driving capacity, the topic is unfamiliar to most physicians and won't easily fit into a brief medical appointment. One helpful set of recommendations urges clinicians to educate patients and family members about the risks of lost financial capacity and to identify warning signs of exploitation.[46] Most clinicians cannot provide a detailed neuropsychological evaluation, but they should refer to a specialist who can.

Unfortunately there is no single simple tool for assessment. Making wise financial choices requires a multitude of skills. You need to have good judgment about who is trustworthy. You need basic math skills. You need to know what is a reasonable price for a thing or service. You need to remember or be able to check whether you've already given to your alumni association three times this year. (Don't laugh: Some schools call elder grads repeatedly for just this reason.) One model includes assessment of cognitive skills, like mental math, as well as social skills, such as the judgment needed to spot a likely scam.[47] This promising approach requires a specialist to administer the test and takes roughly thirty minutes to complete. Those factors will limit accessibility in the short run, but the model has promise for helping protect one's assets.

Financial vulnerability for the elderly is not a new problem—Jonathan Swift's friends tackled this on his behalf in the eighteenth century. The legal system has long offered remedies, particularly through the guardianship process. This approach traditionally required a family to submit an evaluation to a judge, with a request that the person be declared incompetent and that a family member or other trusted person be named guardian, with authority to access all accounts and disburse funds on the person's behalf. Legal scholar and bioethicist Jalayne Arias points out that this approach fails to protect those in the middle, who have neither full capacity nor an utter lack of it.[48] Millions of people with a recent diagnosis, or no diagnosis, of dementia may lose function and assets rapidly before any protections are in place. Arias recommends an intermediate step of limited guardianship that permits some oversight but includes the affected person in financial decision-making on a defined basis.

The Consumer Financial Protection Bureau developed recommendations for the banking industry for staff education and the use of tools to identify unusual banking behavior, like an atypical use of large money orders sent overseas.[49] Joint accounts are one common tool, but easily permit exploitation. They allow another person full access, which lets the joint holder use the incapacitated older person's funds for any purpose. Upon the death of one member of a joint account, the funds are owned wholly by the co-holder, which may exclude other family members from an intended inheritance. Some experts recommend "convenience accounts," from which a designated person can pay bills but will not inherit funds. Other useful tools include "read only" access in which a third party can monitor banking activity and alert the bank about suspicious behavior.[50]

New technical innovations also help. Automatic payment of critical bills, third-party notification of credit card use, and tools that flag risky banking behavior are all available, and more will crop up in coming years. Having relatives you can trust to look after your interests has always been the best plan, though sadly this is not available to us all. Consumer groups, government institutions, and the banking industry are working on it. But so are those who exploit financially vulnerable elders; they will continue to rob vulnerable people of vast amounts, unless we can stop them.

Dementia lasts roughly ten years between diagnosis and the end. That's too much time to just wait for death. We need to think about the decade, not just the last chapter. I want to reflect on where I'll live, who will keep me company, and what makes me happy. Those ten years are not only, not even mostly, about medical treatment. Those years are not about how to die, but about how to live with dementia.

I'd like to find some joy in living with dementia. I want to reflect on my goals and about what is likely to make me happy. I'll build on what I've always liked and try to make those things dementia-friendly. For me, that means adapting reading, walking, and gardening. It's going to take a lot more than that, but that's my start. Reimagining dementia, I hope, will make it more likely for me to hold on to happiness when I get there. And having a more pleasant, less terrifying future to consider helps even today to decrease my dread. To be happy, I'll need to be safe. We haven't done a great job as a society of tackling obvious risks related to sex, driving, and money—and those are just the problems we know about. We'll need to do better. Finding the right balance between freedom and safety is hard in dementia and in life. Looking for sources of joy and watching out for obvious risks start us off on the path to a good life with dementia.

Chapter 12

A Good Ending

Let's play a game. It's not very fun. Even so, millions of Americans are playing it today. The object of the game is to avoid the death you don't want when you die of dementia. There can be multiple winners; there are too many losers. The stakes are high. If you don't play well, you get exactly the wrong death. Some people play because they have risky genes like APOE e4 or a family history. Some already have a diagnosis of minimal cognitive impairment or dementia. A few people play skillfully and look as if they'll do well. Many will lose big; everything they don't want is coming their way. How can you increase the chances of getting what you want and avoiding what you don't want? How do you keep the bad options from ensnaring you once you are too ill and impaired to play anymore? I'll tell you my strategy. If you don't like it, maybe you'll draft one that suits you better.

Medical students are often asked to imagine the ideal death for themselves. The goal is to help them grapple with powerful cultural taboos against thinking or speaking about death, the better for them to deal compassionately with dying patients.[1] Medical students tend to be cheerful little blighters; they imagine colorful ways of heading to the afterlife. Some skydive (not for me). Some put out to sea and drift away on the waters of death. Some construct a Dickensian tableau, a venerable version of themselves in bed at home (with a working fireplace!), devoted family all round, old dog curled at their feet.

The death no one wants is the one we deliver commonly in America: in an intensive care unit, poked by busy worker bees, hooked up to machines and tubes, suffering, tied down, sedated beyond the ability to say goodbye. Older Americans say they'd like to die at home, but 75 percent of people dying in hospitals are over sixty-five.[2] This is the death that awaits a person with dementia—unless she wins the game. To do so, you'll have to be better informed than most. You'll have to be smart about not letting the death you want be derailed by the wishes of others or the entropy of the system. And you'll have to be lucky.

The difference between a good death and a not-so-good death was illustrated in a sadly personal way for me. My parents each died at age eighty-five, though some years apart, and each had hospice care at the end. But my father's death was what he wanted, and my mother's, though not terrible, was not. My father had bladder cancer, and when it was diagnosed, the disease was already beyond cure. He wasn't happy to learn he would die of cancer, but neither was he surprised, nor did he think this a raw deal. He served his country in World War II, then lived a good life and a long one. He had a happy marriage, six children, and fourteen grandchildren. He had been a great poker player in his army days. Now he played the hand he was dealt. He opted for home hospice. At the start, he was in pretty good shape, taking an occasional trip to meet friends for lunch. But time weighed heavy on him. He didn't like waiting. He was not in pain but hated the thought that he might yet be. At the six-month mark he was still around, to his disappointment. He asked me if he should just stop eating, and if I thought the Catholic Church would see this as suicide. He smiled when I pointed out I was not an ideal interpreter of church doctrine—Catholicism having been a topic for epic shouting matches between us in my youth. I observed he was already losing weight fast. The cancer was wasting him away, and wouldn't stop no matter what he ate. What he took in would make little difference in timing and none in the outcome. Why not live it up, enjoying what little food he could? So few pleasures remained to him it seemed a shame to set one aside. He took this approach to heart. One day's intake was a plate of oysters from his favorite raw bar. Another day he had scotch and watermelon, the next a butterscotch sundae. Not too long after that six-month point, my father was gone. He died at home in his own bed. He was comfortable throughout. He was mentally sharp throughout. A lifelong devotee of golf, on his last day he watched a bit of the Masters Tournament and saw Tiger Woods, reputation still unblemished. My father's last words were "the great man." He didn't want to die, but accepted that he must. His death was the one he wanted.

Not so for my mother, who died with hospice care just a few years later. Widowhood plus dementia meant she no longer lived at home. The nursing home sent her repeatedly to the emergency department, unleashing the debate about the unwanted pacemaker. When her status shifted to hospice care, it was because she had declined the pacemaker, not because of her march toward the fatal outcome of dementia. Even when she was on hospice care, nursing home regulations and practice undermined the stockpiling of medications she needed to keep her comfortable at the end. The failure to provide good hospice care meant my mother was not spared one final, uncomfortable, unhelpful transfer from her quiet and comfortable room to a gurney in a noisy, crowded ER. It shouldn't have been that way. Even in hospice care, my mother didn't win the terrible game.

Bad care is the default. We can do better. When people with dementia and their families know more about what's possible and demand it, that creates change. But most important, it's not just that final scene that has to change. Dementia creates a slow decline. The last phase may persist a year or more. It is that whole year we need to fix to arrive at a good death.

What barriers stand between a person with dementia and a good death? For one, people have trouble acknowledging that dementia is fatal. Failure to plan for the inevitable outcome of an illness is a great recipe for not getting the ending you'd like. And it's not just people with dementia or their families who deny that dementia is fatal. The denial is actually recorded in our national death statistics. Thousands of deaths that are listed as caused by pneumonia, infections from bedsores, or other factors are ultimately the result of dementia.[3]

Dementia progresses according to the gloomily named Global Deterioration Scale.[4] The time frame is exceptionally variable; some people move from one phase to the next in only a few months, while others stay in a single phase for years. By definition, it is irreversible. Once a person hits one level of symptoms, he will not go back to a higher level of functioning. It is the final stage, seven, that makes dementia feared more than all illnesses, including AIDS and cancer. Of people in this final phase, roughly 25 percent will die within six months.[5] A person in end-stage dementia cannot walk, may not be able to sit up, or even hold up her head. She may be entirely bedbound, incapable of saying words or understanding them. Incontinence is the norm. Difficulties with swallowing and eating affect almost 90 percent of patients with severe dementia.[6] The capacity to feel pain is as strong as ever, yet it is difficult to identify and treat it in people who can't tell you what the matter is. This is exactly the picture of dementia that frightens us: helpless, in pain, the only relief in death, and that slow in coming.

Curing dementia in this final phase is not a realistic goal—not now, and not later. As far as I know, there is not *any* research for a cure at the end-stage; too many neurons are dead. I have seen families fight for aggressive curative treatment for a person soon to die of dementia; they won't give up on their loved one, and they are sure the right treatment will make her better. Intending no disrespect, I can only say this is not a rational objective. The only possible consequence of medical interventions aimed at a cure in end-stage dementia is more suffering. I don't know what to say when people tell me, "She is a fighter." What I am thinking and cannot say is "Well, that's lucky, because you just put your ninety-four-year-old grandma in the ring with Ali in his prime. How do you think it's going to go?" This is an irreversibly fatal illness, and will remain one. The overwhelming majority of people do not want to extend their life in severe dementia. That doesn't mean people in end-stage dementia need no treatment. They need treatment that relieves suffering. Some would hasten death (more on that later). Comfort should be the goal.

But even hospice may not deliver a good death for those with dementia. Hospice eligibility requires an estimated six-month survival time. Scholars like Joanne Lynn point out that this model is all about cancer, and that it discriminates against those with dementia.[7] Dementia kills just as surely, but more slowly than cancer does. Six months is a reasonable estimate for a death from advanced cancer, but advanced dementia can go on for years and is inherently more unpredictable. For most people, a slow, ineluctable decline, moving only in the direction of loss, is more burdensome than a rapid exit. Hospice can be an acceptable route to the comfortable death, but that route is made rocky by policies that limit the duration of a fatal illness to six months or less. Those policies need to change. Many people on hospice, including those with cancer, outlive that six-month estimate. It is possible to get a patient with severe dementia enrolled in hospice, and re-enroll her six months later. This is today's workaround, as long as the person can re-enroll (no guarantees).

An additional federal policy also stands in the way of hospice care for those in nursing homes, two-thirds of whom have dementia. CMS, which sets Medicare policy, determined that the old regulations increased the enrollment of patients with dementia into hospice. So they changed the rules, offering better compensation for the first few days and less for the remaining period. That effectively works against the use of long-term hospice care, which is appropriate for many with end-stage dementia.[8] But why on earth would you want to keep dying dementia patients off hospice? This change in policy may decrease payments to nursing homes, but will put these patients at greater risk for unhelpful and horribly expensive transfers to hospitals. By financially punishing nursing homes we drive up the overall cost of care *and* provide worse care.

It's possible to be prudent about finances even while striving to offer good care. Accountable Care Organizations (ACOs) are groups of doctors, hospitals, and other health care providers who work together voluntarily to give coordinated high-quality health care to Medicare patients. Right now we rob the starving Paul and pay Peter a bundle for care that doesn't help. Two Health and Aging Policy Scholars recently noted the potential benefits that could come through having Accountable Care Organizations include the hospice benefit; these groups are motivated to consider both the overall cost and value of care across the continuum.[9] Useful policies try to drive us toward high-quality end-of-life care and good value for health care dollars.

Bad policies, ones that fail to envision the larger picture, can drive us off a cliff.

Earlier we looked at how to live with dementia. Now it's time to think about how to die with it. The two tasks are related. Many people are so frightened of the death they don't want that it gets in the way of their living a satisfying life while they can. But let's jump to the finale.

My goals are to avoid bad care and receive good care. Sounds simple, but it's not. By bad care, I mean treatments that will not help me feel better and whose burdens dwarf their benefits. By good care, I mean care that relieves suffering. If I have advanced dementia, I don't want treatments to prolong my life. If a treatment relieves pain but may make my life a little longer, that might be okay, but the main goal is comfort. I do not focus here on cost, but many bad treatments are expensive. (We waste our money on what we don't need and don't want, then can't afford what would help.) If I can avoid them, dying with dementia should be less awful.

I have an advance directive that outlines my treatment preferences. Most of you are familiar with advance directives, though most have not filled one out.[10] For the last thirty years advance directives have been the major tool for guiding your future medical care. They are based on a person's values; they become effective only when the person can no longer make her own decisions. A living will is one type of advance directive. These are if/then statements: If I have condition X, then do or don't do Y to me. Most people use living wills to say what care they don't want when they are near the end of life. The other common advance directive is a proxy or surrogate decision-maker, someone who has the authority to make decisions for you when you are too sick. But for those people who don't formally record their wishes, serious statements to family and friends can also serve as advance directives. We often rely on these spoken records at Montefiore when we work with families to figure out the right thing to do.

I once spoke with a federal health policy maven who asked me with surprise why we need a bioethics consultation service in our hospital. She was under the wildly mistaken impression that having an advance directive neatly resolved decisions at the end of life. Her error is common. You should make an advance directive, but they have serious limitations. Before a new medicine can be prescribed, it undergoes years of testing to prove its safety and efficacy. New public policies rarely get that kind of rigorous examination before they're unleashed on the public. Enormous efforts that encourage the creation of advance directives have succeeded in the sense that more people now dutifully fill out the forms. But the truth is, they just don't work that well.[11] Please don't take my criticism as a reason to put it off altogether: you should have an advance directive. But realize that a living will won't get you all that close to winning the game.

Advance directives have structural flaws. The main ingredients are you, your surrogate decision-makers, and your health providers; any one of you can cause trouble. Let's talk about you first. You are trying to predict what treatment you would want in a condition you're not in. Maybe you know a lot about what's coming your way and have thought about the options; maybe not so much. If you have end-stage lung disease and have been on a ventilator many times, you have well-informed views about that particular treatment. But most of us see through a glass darkly, guessing at what threatens us and what responses exist. If there are any questions about what you want when the time comes, it will be tough to ask you. If you could tell us, you wouldn't need to use the advance directive. So be careful what you wish for. An advance directive is a rough guide, a summary of your views. It can't make things happen; it's not a magic wand. If you tell your children never to put you in a nursing home, make sure you've left close to a million dollars for them to carry out that wish—*after* you've lived off your retirement funds for twenty-five years. And if you don't want to suffer, even if that might mean forgoing some treatments, make sure your family knows that.

Surrogate decision-makers can also create hurdles between you and the care you want. When you appoint a loved one to make decisions for you, you may pick exactly the person who will have the hardest time letting you go. The surrogate is told to make decisions based on *your* values and wishes, not on what they would choose. That can be a tall order for a spouse of sixty years, who cannot imagine life without you. Still, a surrogate who cares about you is better than one who does not. A person who doesn't know your values, who is less likely to feel your pain, will make different and worse mistakes. So we rely on family members, either appointed or not, to make decisions for you when you are too ill to make them yourself.

Bioethicists have written lots about the difficulty of interpreting advance directives. Suppose you hate the idea of yourself with dementia. You ask that if you reach a state in which you don't know your loved ones and can't function at the level you'd like, you want to decline all lifesaving treatments. But when you actually get to that state, you are a cute old person, sitting happily in your chair, rocking, humming, and eating peanut butter and jelly sandwiches. You can't do the things you used to do, but you don't seem unhappy. Should we work to continue this life, which your former self loathed but your current self seems to enjoy, more or less?[12] Having sat through conversations on this topic for decades of my professional life, I conclude it's no longer a useful argument. Bioethicists view this as a problem of identity; the person who wrote the directive is not the person in the chair. While that may be true, it's not relevant. This is a problem of efficacy. The person happily humming in the rocker doesn't need life-sustaining treatment. When she does, she has fallen critically ill within the context of dementia, a fatal illness. The chances of saving her life, even with intensive care, are poor. And if you do save her from a critical illness—say, a serious pneumonia—she will recover slowly if at all. In particular, her fragile cognitive function will take a serious, likely irremediable hit. She may never return to the chair and her humming, and she'll fall ill again more readily. What did she ever do to you that you would doom her to a final year in and out of the ICU? Even if she had not completed an advance directive, her family needs to know that the burdens of many treatments for her outweigh the benefits. That doesn't mean we should ignore her. What she needs is palliative care. If I am ever this woman, keep me comfortable where I am. No hospital, no ventilator, no pain.

Families and doctors can interpret advance directives differently from each other and from what you wanted. It might say, "If I no longer recognize my family members, I do not want cardiac resuscitation." But what if your daughter visits you every day and believes you still recognize her? Does that mean you should not have a do-not-resuscitate (DNR) order? Or what if you have a DNR order, but you get pneumonia? The nursing home sends you to the ER, and in the ER they put you on a breathing tube, which means now they have to send you up to intensive care. That ICU stay will not make you comfortable. Your heart never stopped, so there was no attempt to resuscitate you, but this may be exactly the type of care you didn't want. No one set out to ignore your wishes, but step by step they did. This is a big part of the problem. The default is more treatment. If there is doubt about the right thing to do, more treatment. If there is no one to say stop, more treatment. If no one consents to hospice for you, more treatment. Will this cure your underlying illness or improve your life's quality? Not if you have advanced dementia, but you'll get more treatment anyway.

Some people try to improve upon the living will by making it a mini-compendium of all medical treatments. This is not an effective strategy. Before the ink is dry there will be a new treatment not on the list. The better approach is to focus on goals of treatment, rather than on the specific treatments themselves. The mantra of our bioethics consultation service, articulated by my colleague, Dr. Hannah I. Lipman, is *goals, not interventions*. An advance directive is a guide to the person's values; it is not a contract, in which anything not nailed down is up for grabs. If the living will indicates the person does not want a prolonged dying process, that is the message we should take. Dialysis may not be listed, but if the gist is "keep me comfortable as my time approaches," then dialysis need not be part of the program.

Despite all these caveats, I have set up advance directives, including a proxy. I will increase the odds of success by speaking with my family. If you don't have a family or someone willing to serve as a surrogate, then an advance directive can be especially important. When no one knows your wishes, you are likely to get more treatment, whether it has a good chance of success or not. New York State, like most states, has a form available to fill out. I can decline specific treatments for when I am terminally ill, in a coma, or permanently unable to make decisions. In that condition, I don't want cardiopulmonary resuscitation, mechanical ventilation, artificial nutrition or hydration, or antibiotics. The form doesn't ask about hospitalization, but I'll add that to my list. I'd rather be kept as comfortable as possible wherever I am. Transfers back and forth from home or nursing home to ER to hospital are a major source of suffering at the end of life; that is one of the main things I don't want in that final year.[13]

The treatments I decline epitomize bad care for someone in severe dementia. Let's think about resuscitation, or the attempt to restart my heart if it should stop. The chances of restarting my heart when I have end-stage dementia are minimal. I don't want treatment that doesn't help but can still cause pain! Because resuscitation is worse for someone with severe dementia in the unlikely case that it works. I will likely have painfully broken ribs, and my brain will have been further damaged from going without oxygen while my heart wasn't working. Resuscitation attempts maximize the possibility of suffering for those in end-stage dementia.

I don't want a breathing tube either. Patients sometimes wind up with these due to poor communication from doctors. And here is where I get to the third group of players who can undermine your advance directive. Doctors have a lot to learn about communication. We are not good at delivering bad news. This is embarrassing to admit, since that's been part of our job description these last few thousand years. The advent of palliative care inspired a wave of efforts to study and improve physician communication, but there is still a lot of room for improvement.[14] A doctor might say, "There's a chance your mother could recover from her pneumonia if we put her on the breathing tube and send her to the ICU." A chance? That sounds great! A more accurate statement might be something like this: "We could put your mother in the ICU on a breathing tube. I don't recommend that, because she will suffer, without likely benefit. The tube is so uncomfortable she will have to be sedated, so she can't communicate with you. She may get restrained so she doesn't pull out the tube. If she gets through this pneumonia, she will be weaker than before, and more likely to get sick again. This pneumonia signals she is in the final phase of dementia. I recommend that you consider hospice care and a do-not-hospitalize order, focusing on comfort care without the pain and trauma of repeated transfers as she grows weaker." A family member will have a clearer picture of how this treatment fits into the larger scenario of old age, dementia, and frailty. Better communication about outcomes and the overall picture helps families limit a loved one's suffering before death.

Feeding tubes are bad care for people with severe dementia. They are also common, and it's easy to see why. Difficulties with swallowing are the norm in end-stage dementia, affecting over 90 percent of patients. Geriatricians and palliative care specialists have battled against the use of feeding tubes in severe dementia for decades, but the problem continues for several reasons. First, few patients or their family members realize what symptoms emerge as dementia unfolds. The Alzheimer's Association and other groups have tried hard to make accurate information available, but surprisingly many family members remain astonished at the predictable symptoms of dementia, including problems with swallowing and eating. Second, not only are family members and patients poorly informed about swallowing problems, they know even less about potential responses. It might sound like a feeding tube could help a person with dementia and trouble swallowing, but that's false. A feeding tube in severe dementia neither extends life nor improves its quality.[15] It can increase agitation, since it's uncomfortable, and the likelihood of bedsores, since the tube makes it harder to accomplish the frequent re-positioning that is crucial to prevent bed-sores, which greatly increase the risk of infection and death in this highly vulnerable group. This is bad treatment.

An array of perverse incentives encourages the use of feeding tubes, and few families know enough to push back. For a long time nursing homes objected to caring for patients who could not feed themselves and lacked a feeding tube. An aide would have to carefully hand-feed each severely demented person, and this care took too much staff time.

(Translation: Time is money.) Nursing homes would send patients to the hospital to have a feeding tube inserted and would refuse to take them back without a tube. Informed consent was a sham. A gastroenterologist would get consent by saying to the family, "Your mother can't swallow anymore. She has to have a feeding tube or she will die." That sounds pretty compelling, and when the conversation goes this way, most families consent. The problem is the fundamental dishonesty of such a description. A person with severe dementia and difficulty swallowing will die. She has a fatal illness. There is no "or she will die." A feeding tube does not prevent choking or the infections that can result when a person gets secretions from the esophagus in the breathing passage. Nor is it correct to say the person will starve to death without the tube. The choice is not between starvation and food; it is between feeding someone by hand, accommodating their disability, and administering mush through a tube directly to the stomach. The processed food for the tube is expensive, but the nursing home gets well reimbursed for that, so they don't object. The doctor gets paid to insert the tube, and thus may not object either. The person with dementia never again tastes real food, one of the last remaining pleasures for a person with advanced dementia, and loses an opportunity for direct and caring human contact several times daily.

A better discussion would be more like this: "Your mother now has difficulty swallowing, a symptom of end-stage dementia. In the past, we used to give feeding tubes to patients like your mother, but we no longer recommend that. Feeding tubes don't make life longer, and they make the quality of remaining time worse. She may still get pleasure from eating, and we'd like her to have that as long as possible. We'll shift to careful hand-feeding, with foods she likes that are easier to swallow. Many of our patients with severe dementia love milk shakes, and we'll try that. If you'd like to help feed her we can train you—a lot of family members enjoy this way of being close as the illness progresses." This is comfort feeding, in which the person is offered food she likes, designed to be delicious and easy to swallow. (The time to worry about cholesterol is over.) As the dementia progresses, the person will eat less, both because he or she has difficulty swallowing and because appetite vanishes in those who are dying. Comfort feeding dwindles based on what the person can tolerate. When someone is in the last few days of life, that may be only sips of water, or even just enough fluid to prevent the mouth from feeling dry.

Efforts to end the use of feeding tubes in advanced dementia are gaining ground. The American Board of Internal Medicine put together a project called Choosing Wisely, in which different medical specialties develop lists of common treatments to avoid because they don't benefit patients. The geriatricians' list of ten treatments to avoid, in the top position, states: "Don't recommend percutaneous feeding tubes in patients with advanced dementia; instead offer oral assisted feeding."[16] This high-profile recommendation broadcasts that feeding tubes do more harm than good, but it won't stop their use altogether. The gastroenterologists who insert the tube have no such recommendation on their Choosing Wisely list. Still, the tide is changing. More nursing homes provide hand-feeding as part of efforts to improve end-of-life dementia care. Some facilities train volunteers to do hand-feeding, offering a way to unite the compassion of visitors with the dementia patient's need for human contact. For me, no feeding tube.

There is a further step you could take. Some people create an advance directive to stop all food and fluid by mouth when their dementia advances to a certain point. Most living wills offer the option of refusing invasive feeding (as through a feeding tube) and hydration, and this is not the same. Neither is this the same as requesting comfort feeding, which naturally decreases with a dying person's tolerance for food. This option is to take someone who remains capable of swallowing and still eating, and no longer offering them food and fluid by mouth. For me, this is too far, but not everyone agrees. Paul Mendel and Colette Chandler-Cramer argue for an advance directive that tells nursing home staff to withhold food and fluid when a person reaches a specified stage of dementia, such as not recognizing their family.[17] They acknowledge that problems arise if a person with such an advance directive still enjoys eating, and they would ignore the advance directive if the person still wants to eat when the previously listed stage occurs. They would honor the advance directive and stop food and fluid if the person actively refuses food or merely seems indifferent.

I don't see the benefit of abruptly stopping food and fluid, as opposed to comfort feeding, which gradually diminishes with the person's capacity to swallow. This also sounds like a recipe for moral distress in the nursing staff. The fear of liability and the regulatory burdens are great for nursing homes, and these directives would be hard to honor. Still, a family needs only one nursing home to agree. Or this approach could work for a person cared for by family on home hospice. If your family is very clear about your wishes and willing to carry them out, this plan could work and no one else might ever know. Not everyone would be comfortable doing this, but you just need your family to agree.

As I said, I prefer comfort feeding; it offers all the benefits and none of the drawbacks. I'd like to have a chance for the few pleasures available at the end. I think back to my father's death, and how happy it made him to still taste his favorite foods. The amount I'll eat when my dementia is severe is unlikely to prolong my time. People who don't want life prolonged in the final phase should make sure they don't get ventilators, resuscitation, feeding tubes, or other unhelpful treatment, like transitions from the nursing home to the emergency department to the hospital and back again. Treatment should focus on comfort. If we just did that, we'd go a long way toward improving that final phase of dementia. And your granddaughter could still feed you a last bit of apple pie.

For any treatment, ask if it will increase comfort right now, not after a flogging in the ICU. Watch out for doctors who say of a person near the end of a fatal illness, "She has to have X or she'll die." The person you are talking about is going to die, no way out. The question is how, and whether this treatment is likely to get this person closer to the death she hopes for. And watch out for doctors who say, "No one should die of X." What that generally means is that X can be treated, not that it's a bad way to go. If a person is dying, focus on comfort and stop trying to prevent it. Death from dementia is slow and not especially desirable. Death from many other things, if they are on offer, may be better.

What about speeding the process up? What about physician aid in dying, also known as physician-assisted suicide? Bad news: All U.S. states with legalized physician aid in dying require the person to be fully capable of making a rational decision, and to have six months or less to live. If you have advanced dementia, you won't qualify because you lack decisional capacity. If you have early stage dementia, you won't qualify because you have more than six months to live. I see no prospect of a law passing in the United States that would support aid in dying for those with severe dementia. The four states that have passed aid in dying laws all use variants of the same model bill, which succeeded in part because they *exclude* those with cognitive disabilities. This issue activates the third rail in U.S. politics, the one attached to abortion. Our entrenched battles mean that any issue connected with the right to life galvanizes passionate support from both sides of our unbridgeable cultural divide. You may find that everyone you know agrees with you on this issue, but that is because our communities are divided along fault lines. Even most supporters do not want to add an option for those with cognitive impairment, since that could derail the project of promoting aid in dying in the remaining states. And those who object are particularly distressed by the slippery slope argument, that assisted dying would start with clear-thinking people and rapidly progress to killing off anyone who is imperfect. Aid in dying for those with dementia is not coming any sooner than a cure. We will still need to work on figuring out how to provide and pay for good care and fend off bad care.

Some plan to beat dementia with the old-fashioned DIY approach to suicide. Suicide looms before anyone who lives and suffers; it has always been there and always will be. As a psychiatrist, I have worked with people who struggled against suicide. We would look for ways to buy time, to see what would help them tolerate or diminish pain, to see what we could change that might help. With luck, creativity, and great courage, some people overcome the lure of suicide and build satisfying lives. You may say that this battle just can't be won with dementia. I don't think we've done the work to support that conclusion. Suicide is a blunt tool for the relief of suffering. We need to do a lot more to support a good life and a good death. We are nowhere near saying that we have done all we could to relieve suffering from dementia and that hastening death is the only respite.

I hate the idea of suicide as the best response to dementia we as a society can offer. I respect that some people will prefer this exit. But I don't want it to be door number one. A philosopher argued a few years ago in the *American Journal of Bioethics* that people with dementia have a moral obligation to kill themselves.[18] Not an option; an obligation. I coauthored a response with the late Adrienne Asch, noteworthy bioethicist and advocate for the disabled; it was the angriest essay I've ever written.[19] The original author assumed, without examination, that a life with dementia is a life without dignity. This caught my attention, since my mother then had dementia and enjoyed a comfortable, even dignified, existence. But no, this author felt the demented should be ashamed that they are no longer at cognitive top form, and do us all a favor by offing themselves. Adrienne and I were upset even before he praised the classical example of women who killed themselves because rape made them worthless. That pretty much put us around the bend. Not knowing of Swift's connection to dementia, we based the response on his "Modest Proposal." Why wait for suicide? we asked. Why not go ahead and kill those with dementia, and indeed all the disabled? And why not then eat them, killing two undesirable birds with one stone?

One more word on suicide: It's hard to get things done when you are cognitively impaired, and that applies to suicide in dementia. If you end your life while you are capable, you miss some good times. If you wait, you won't have the skills. The title character in Lisa Genova's *Still Alice* has such a plan (spoiler alert), which fails miserably because of her increasing disability. Real-life people have the same plan, and some succeed.[20] I don't judge. I also fear severe dementia. I hope to deal with my fear by preserving as much of the good in life for as long as possible. When I reach dementia's end-stage, I'd be delighted if pneumonia or another speedy, relatively painless illness swept me away. In part my reservations about suicide come from observing the devastation left behind for survivors. I concede it is awful to watch a loved person linger at the edge of death. We need to do a better job of making sure people don't suffer at the end or during any part of that final year or more. Some may choose to end their lives because of dementia, but it shouldn't be because they can't get good care.

I've talked about bad care. What does good care look like? It is an extension of moral treatment; it is palliative care, focused on comfort. (Hospice is care at the end of life, which includes palliative care, but palliative care is broader and promotes comfort at any stage of life.) An innovative model of palliative care specifically for people with dementia comes from the Beatitudes Campus in Phoenix, Arizona.[21] It is not just for the final year; it can start earlier and continue until the end. Caregivers here ease up on a lot of rules typical of nursing homes. They allow patients to sleep and get up as it suits them; they ignore a lot of dietary restrictions; they don't use physical restraints and they use much less "chemical restraint" in the form of drugs for psychosis and anxiety. Though they use fewer drugs overall, they use more drugs for pain, as they find pain is a common, often undiagnosed, reason for agitation. The goal is to think broadly of ways to increase comfort. Understandably, patients are happier with this regimen, but their families are also far more satisfied with the care their loved ones receive, and there is markedly less staff turnover.[22]

Consider how this approach worked for ND, a patient who spent much of each day yelling and lived at a New York nursing home adapting the Beatitudes approach.[23] This is the kind of behavior that has long made nursing homes terrifying for other patients and visiting relatives and enervating for staff. Typical responses would be restraint, sedation, and moving the (still yelling) patient out of the way so no one need hear her. None of that helps the person or fixes what is troubling her. The staff there met and brainstormed together. Perhaps there was too much stimulation in the dayroom, or maybe having a personal aide by her side was agitating rather than calming her? The staff moved ND so she could see the dayroom but was somewhat sheltered from the commotion there; they spoke to her family, who agreed to withdraw the personal attendant. Both these interventions helped for a time. When the yelling resumed, the staff did more troubleshooting, shifting her location throughout the day, playing opera on her iPod, and giving pain medication. The patient grew calmer; the staff kept thinking about what more they could do to keep her comfortable. That is what good palliative care, specifically designed for dementia, looks like.

When, in the context of dementia, is it right to shift the balance away from curative care to palliative care? It is wrong to deny treatment for reversible illness to someone diagnosed yesterday with minimal cognitive impairment. But it is cruel to load invasive treatment onto someone for whom there is no realistic expectation of recovery or benefit. I've often wondered about the relative risks and burdens of my mother's hospitalizations during dementia. Her first hospitalization made sense. She was quite chipper about life; she enjoyed walking as much as a mile a day. She knew her family. She loved her grandchildren and little kids generally. She fed herself and would tell anyone how much she loved sweets. Treating her first acute medical illness to see if she could get back to baseline was right. When her dementia had progressed further, we were correct to refuse her pacemaker. I'll never forgive her cardiologist for the abusive line "No one is allowed to die from heart block." When people die asleep in their beds at night, this is often what they die from. This is exactly the way you want to go. Preventing that exit for someone who is old and frail and will die within the next year is cruel.

I don't expect to get through life without any disability. I have depended on others in one way or another all my life. That's part of the human condition and nothing to be ashamed of. I agree with those who find us too caught up in cognitive abilities as a measure of personhood.[24] Being cognitively intact is an important part of my identity, as it is for most of us. But if I develop dementia, I'll have significant deficits before I'm done. Disability will be my lot. That's not what I worry about most.

What I worry about is pain and suffering. Every intervention should lead to comfort. I do not want to extend my life in severe dementia. I do not want a ventilator, even temporarily. I don't want a feeding tube. No pacemaker, no implantable defibrillator. If I can swallow and seem to enjoy food, offer me tasty bites. Don't fuss with a balanced diet or adequate calories. If I can have a tiny piece of dark chocolate on my tongue, why shouldn't I have it? Don't send me to the hospital unless it is the only way to make me comfortable. I will be way past medical screening, like colonoscopies or mammograms. If I get cancer, stick with comfort care. I don't want antibiotics. Keep me comfortable, and don't stand between me and the exit.

That's what I want for the final phase. I'm guessing that might be year ten. A lot of planning needs to go into the decade before that. I don't want to bankrupt my family or ruin my children's lives. My husband and I don't know who's going first, but if he's around for my disability, I'd like it to go as easily on him as possible. I'd like to stay home as long as that's affordable and convenient. That will mean getting cost-effective help, to give him a break and help keep me out of an institution. I'd be happy to go to a day program where I have lunch with my cronies, get my blood pressure checked, sing badly (the only option for me), and do chair yoga. When I have moderate dementia, maybe technology can help me stay home without an expensive full-time helper. I picture a granny cam linked to a call center with a worker who calls a mobile unit in case of emergency, like a person stuck on the floor who can't get up. To keep me safe, you might need to turn off the stove and other appliances. I hope no one has to stay in my house overnight just because I have a disturbed sleep-wake cycle. It's expensive care and not great for the worker or the patient. We won't have enough caregivers to go around. I'd like to see us pay them better and employ them more efficiently. If robots can do some jobs, fine with me. If we use technology appropriately, we can extend the time during which people with dementia can safely and affordably stay home.

I see these plans taking me through several years of dementia, on my own or with my aging husband. As I get frailer, I may need more care than a day program can reasonably provide. If I can't stay home but don't qualify for a nursing home, my family will need to consider assisted living. Some long-term care policies cover assisted living; Medicaid does in some states but not in all. The cost of care varies by location to an absurd extent. One site estimated the *monthly* cost of living at home with a full-time home health aide in New York City at nearly $14,000. In contrast, assisted living averaged $6,500 per month. In a rural area of New York State, assisted living went down to $4,000 monthly, while an attendant cost a shocking $17,000 monthly.[25] If a person needs additional help in assisted living, that can raise costs considerably. I want to avoid bankrupting my family. Staying home may not be the way to do that.

Like nursing homes, assisted living facilities are as variable as their costs. A detailed analysis would take a book, and there are some helpful ones on the topic.[26] When considering assisted living, my main advice is to ignore the chandelier. That is for family members, so they don't feel they're sending mom to the pit of despair. Instead, look at how people live. Can they sleep and wake on their own schedule, or do they get roused rudely out of bed as in jail? Can they eat when they want, or will they miss breakfast if they don't get up on the facility's schedule? Some of the best places are not glamorous, but manage to create a real sense of community. If I go to assisted living, I'd like to stay there as I decline, and some places make that impossible. Others embrace the likelihood of change, by offering different levels of care, including palliative care and hospice on site. I want to avoid the cycle of transfer from where I live, whether at home or in a facility, back and forth to the emergency department, the hospital, and home again.

Going to the ED can only exacerbate pain; it makes no sense at all. Emergency departments serve incredibly important purposes, but providing comfort care at the end of life is not one of them. I'd like to maximize care I can get at home, wherever that is, and if I can't get it there, maybe I don't need it. Good pain control is where I started, and that's where I'll end. By the time I need it, I hope there will be lots of roving units that address pain for people at home and in nursing homes and assisted living facilities. There are a few of these now, but not nearly enough. If the rules change, I may more easily qualify for hospice than is possible now, but even now I would hope for competent palliative care throughout my experience of dementia.

You may not want what I want. You may want lots of medical care toward the end, though most people don't. You may want even less than I do, and you may want to stop eating and drinking altogether. Whatever you want, though, is not what you'll get unless you plan realistically and carefully. Find out about the symptoms of dementia and talk to your children about your values. Talk to your doctor. Make sure you write down your preferences, since medicine is changing fast and we have no way of knowing who your doctor will be in five years.

I don't want to die badly. I want treatment for pain. I'll ask my family to help ward off the interventions piled on people who can't defend themselves. My family and doctors will know what I want. Hell, even *you* will know what I want. Now decide what you want, based on what's available, and make that clear to your family and doctors. Maybe we'll all win this game.

None of us knows what kind of ending we're in for. Still, to paraphrase Damon Runyon, though the race is not always to the swift nor the battle to the strong, that is definitely the way to bet. I bet

I'll develop dementia. I admit this thought makes me sad. I have benefited so much from education; it is my greatest wealth. My little flock
of facts and ideas will vanish over time, quietly, stolen one by one by
the wolf of dementia. I won't see them going, so I'll say goodbye now.
Goodbye, imaginary friends, residing in your well-loved books: *Middle-
march*'s Dorothea Brook, Lady Glencora, Elizabeth Bennet, Jack
Aubrey, and Stephen Maturin. Goodbye to Elizabeth Bishop, subject
of my college thesis, and your artful losing. Goodbye, psychiatry, bioethics, and the best terrible jokes of my father and father-in-law; goodbye to the *Saturday Night Live* cork soakers clip. Music lasts longer,
so I hope I'll long be happy to hear "Let's Groove." As memory goes,
I'll lose people. Goodbye, students, patients, colleagues. Goodbye, my
dearest friends, my family, even my husband and children. I'll bet that
even if someday I don't know you, I'll see in your faces great beauty.

Even toward the end I hope still to have some joy. I may not get
there, but I'd like to see again one of my old familiar places: the dancing world of Central Park on a perfect day. Leaves shimmer overhead
in a light breeze. Midair Frisbees fly while dogs and people arc grace-
fully up to seize them from the ether. On the ground a young couple
on a picnic blanket, Motown on their boombox. Their wobbly first
child stands, resplendent in a dinosaur-print onesie, his small hands in
the large ones of his seated father. He cannot walk yet, but he dances,
bobbing his padded bottom up and down. His face is the portrait of
happiness, with the sun, his parents' love, the breeze, the music all
radiating through him. If I could be there again, trees, breeze, flying
dogs, and dancing babies, that would be enough. I'll be seeing you.

Acknowledgments

So many people helped create this book that I hardly know where to start giving thanks. I choose to begin with the experts on dementia who participated in interviews, and who were candid, even brave, in thinking out loud about this illness and what to do about it. These generous scholars and clinicians include (alphabetically): Mirnova Ceide, Dan Cohen, Tara Cortes, Peter Davies, Nancy Dubler, Amy Ehrlich, David Hoffman, T. Byram Karasu, Gary Kennedy, Zaven Khachaturian, Carol Levine, Jed Levine, Joann Lynn, Mary Mittelman, Richard Mayeux, Dominic Ruscio, Sandy Selikson, Sharon Shaw, Reisa Sperling, Yaakov Stern, Lynn Street, Rick Surpin, Joe Verghese, Bruce Vladeck, and Kristine Yaffe. Many friends and colleagues read versions of the book and offered invaluable advice; these include Cathy Cramer, Monica Dolin, Amy Ehrlich, Katie Geisinger, Ken Gibbs, Donald Margulies, Kathy Pike, JillEllyn Riley, Jim Shapiro, Aiden Shapiro, Billy Shebar, and John Thornton. I am very lucky that my dear friend Lynn Street, geriatrician and former editor, and my colleague Gary Kennedy, geriatric psychiatrist, were indefatigable and knowledgeable readers who pored over drafts and offered detailed notes and critical insights. I benefited from a capable editorial team in Megan Newman, Nina Shield, and Hannah Steigmeyer. The book would not be what it is without the thoughtful comments of these readers.

During my year with the Health and Aging Policy Fellowship I was on a steep learning curve, and am grateful for the wisdom of the other fellows, colleagues in Health and Human Services, in the Office of the Assistant Secretary for Planning and Evaluation and at NIH. Colleagues on the Board of Isabella Geriatric Center and at CaringKind have improved my understanding of the challenges of caring for those with dementia. I appreciate the competence and professionalism of library staff at both the Katzman Archives, Special Collections and Archives, University of California–San Diego, and the Schomburg Center for Research in Black Culture, New York Public Library. Dominic Ruscio offered access to his personal papers from the early years of Alzheimer lobbying, even lending me a number of documents. The Montefiore Einstein Center for Bioethics sponsors undergraduate summer interns each year, and they have provided invaluable assistance for my academic courses and this book, delighting in the antique articles of the *American Journal of Insanity*, checking footnotes, and generally offering their keen minds and youthful enthusiasm. These research assistants include Beverly Adade, Annabel Barry, Emma Brezel, Alexa Kanbergs, Alicia Lai, Rachel Linfield, David Meister, Madeline Russell, and Beau Sperry. I am especially grateful to my supervisors, Andrew Racine and Ed Burns, for a crucial six-month sabbatical that permitted me to work full-time on the book. I have learned from countless other colleagues, especially at Montefiore Health System and Albert Einstein College of Medicine and within the Montefiore Einstein Center for Bioethics. Each has enriched my understanding, though all errors are surely my own.

I must thank another group of experts to whom I am immensely indebted, though I will not identify them by name. These are involuntary experts in dementia, those who either have the illness or care for someone who does, and who have shared their stories with me. I have removed identifying information from their accounts and substituted some details in ways that leave the essential narrative intact, yet these remain the stories of very real people. As a physician, the knowledge I have to share with others is embedded in what I have learned from patients and their family members. I cannot tell you what I know without telling you what I learned from them, and yet I feel keenly the obligation to protect their privacy and respect the courage of their contributions.

I thank my family. In sharing stories about my parents and childhood, I tread upon the stories of my five brothers and sisters, and know full well they might have chosen to tell these stories differently or not at all. I am grateful for their trust. My two adult children give me great joy, as they have from the start, and provide much of the fuel that keeps me going. Finally, I thank my husband, Jim Shapiro. His kindness, his unwavering confidence in me, and his awful jokes make me laugh and make me happy to be alive.

Notes

CHAPTER 1. DE-'MEN-SHA: AN INTRODUCTION

1 Tia Powell, "Voice: Cognitive Impairment and Medical Decision Making." *Journal of Clinical Ethics* 16.4 (2005): 303–13.
2 *2017 Alzheimer's Disease Facts and Figures.* Alzheimer's Association, 2017. alz.org /documents_custom/2017-facts-and-figures.pdf.
3 Michael D. Hurd et al., "Monetary Costs of Dementia in the United States." *New England Journal Medicine* 368.14 (2013): 1326–34.
4 Ibid.
5 John Hancock, 2016 Cost of Care Survey; Long Term Care Insurance. ubsnet.com /assets/Uploads/Newspdf/2016-LTC-Cost-of-Care-Survey-Results.pdf.
6 Tia Powell, "Life Imitates Work." *JAMA* 305.6 (2011): 542–43.

CHAPTER 2. INVISIBLE

1 Cited in Leo Damrosch, *Jonathan Swift: His Life & His World.* New Haven: Yale University Press, 2013.
2 See, for instance, Will Durant and Ariel Durant, *The Story of Civilization: The Age of Reason Begins, 1558–1648.* Vol. VII. New York: Simon & Schuster, 1961.
3 Damrosch, *Jonathan Swift: His Life & His World.*
4 Jonathan Swift, Letter to Mrs. Whiteaway, July 26, 1740, quoted in Damrosch, *Jonathan Swift: His Life & His World,* 466, note 40.
5 Quoted in Damrosch, *Jonathan Swift: His Life & His World,* 466, note 41.
6 Ibid., 467, note 43.
7 *Diagnostic and Statistical Manual of Mental Disorders,* 5th ed. (*DSM-5*). Arlington, VA: American Psychiatric Association, 2013.

8 "Global Aging," *National Institute on Aging*. U.S. Department of Health and Human Services; nia.nih.gov/research/dbsr/global-aging.

9 Aretaeus, *The Extant Works of Aretæus, the Cappadocian*. Ed. and trans. Francis Adams. London: Sydenham Society, 1856.

10 B. Mahendra, *Dementia: A Survey of the Syndrome of Dementia*. Lancaster, UK: MTP Press Limited; 1987, quoted in N. C. Berchtold and C. W. Cotman, "Evolution in the Conceptualization of Dementia and Alzheimer's Disease: Greco-Roman Period to the 1960s." *Neurobiology of Aging* 19.3 (1998): 173–89.

11 Juvenal, 10.232–35, (trans P. Green), cited in Karen Cokayne, *Experiencing Old Age in Ancient Rome*. London and New York: Routledge, 2003, 70.

12 Cokayne, *Experiencing Old Age*, 192, note 57.

13 Daniel Hack Tuke, *Chapters in the History of the Insane in the British Isle*. London: Kegan Paul, Trench & Co., 1882; reprint Whitefish, MT: Kessinger Publishing, 2009, 20.

14 For a fuller discussion of this era in the history of mental illness, see Gerald N. Grob, *Mental Illness and American Society, 1875–1940*. Princeton, NJ: Princeton University Press, 1983.

15 Museo Ebraico di Venezia [Jewish Museum of Venice], "The Ghetto," museoebraico.it/en/ghetto/.

16 David J. Rothman, *The Discovery of the Asylum: Social Order and Disorder in the New Republic*, 2nd ed. London and New York: Routledge, 2002.

17 Edward A. Strecker, "Reminiscences from the Early Days of the Pennsylvania Hospital." *American Journal of Psychiatry* 88.5 (March 1932): 972–79.

18 Ibid.

19 William L. Russell, "A Psychopathic Department of an American General Hospital in 1808." *American Journal of Psychiatry* 98.2 (September 1941): 229–37.

20 Ibid.

21 Benjamin Rush, *Medical Inquiries and Observations Upon the Diseases of the Mind*. Philadelphia: Kimber and Richardson, 1812. U.S. National Library of Medicine Digital Collections, nlm.nih.gov/catalog/nlm:nlmuid-2569036R-bk.

22 Ibid., 35, 372.

23 Ibid., 342.

24 Ibid., 296.

25 Jonathan Andrews, Asa Briggs, Roy Porter, Penny Tucker, and Keir Waddington, *The History of Bethlem*. London & New York: Routledge, 1997, 421.

26 Unsigned review of *Chapters in the History of the Insane in the British Isles*. *American Journal of Insanity* 39.2 (1882), 239.

27 Ibid. See p. 253.

28 Henry Viets, "A Note from Samuel Tuke to the New York Hospital (1811)." *American Journal of Psychiatry* 78.3 (1922): 425–32.

29 John B. Chapin, "Dr. Thomas Story Kirkbride: An Address on the Presentation of His Portrait to the College of Physicians, Philadelphia, January 5, 1898." *American Journal of Insanity* 55 (1898): 119–29.

30 Thomas Kirkbride, *Code of Rules and Regulations for the Government of Those Employed in the Care of the Patients of the Pennsylvania Hospital for the Insane, near Philadelphia*. Philadelphia: T. K. and P. G. Collins, 1850, 31. U.S. National Library of Medicine Digital Collections, resource.nlm.nih.gov/101560452.

31 Kirkbride, quoted in Rothman, *The Discovery of the Asylum,* 148.

32 Orpheus Everts, "The American System of Public Provision for the Insane, and Despotism in Lunatic Asylums." *American Journal of Insanity* 38.2 (1881): 113–39.

CHAPTER 3. THE BIG HOUSE: ITS RISE AND FALL

1 Dorothea Dix, *Memorial, to the Legislature of Massachusetts,* 1843. U.S. National Library of Medicine Digital Collections, resource.nlm.nih.gov/7703963.

2 Clarence O. Cheney, "Dorothea Lynde Dix: Servant of the Lord." *American Journal of Psychiatry* 100.6 (1944): 60–62.

3 Manon S. Parry, "Dorothea Dix (1802–1887)." *American Journal of Public Health* 96.4 (2006): 624–25.

4 Cheney, "Dorothea Dix."

5 New-York Hospital. "Address of the Governors of the New-York Hospital, to the public: relative to the Asylum for the Insane at Bloomingdale." New York, May 1821. U.S. National Library of Medicine Digital Collections, resource.nlm.nih.gov/68130900R.

6 Ibid.

7 Earl Bond, "A Mental Hospital in the 'Fabulous Forties.'" *American Journal of Psychiatry* 81.3 (1925): 527–36.

8 "Address of the Governors of the New-York Hospital," 1821, 10.

9 *Report of the Commissioners Appointed under a Resolve of the Legislature of Massachusetts to Superintend the Erection of a Lunatic Hospital at Worcester and to Report a System of Discipline and Government for the Same.* Boston: Dutton and Wentworth, 1832. Signed by Commissioners Horace Mann, Bezaleel Taft Jr., and W. B. Calhoun.

10 *Report of the Commissioners,* 38.

11 Gerald N. Grob, *Mental Illness and American Society, 1875–1940.* Princeton, NJ: Princeton University Press, 1987, 76.

12 Worcester Insane Asylum, *Eleventh Annual Report of the Trustees of the Worcester Insane Asylum at Worcester, for the Year Ending September 30, 1888,* Forgotten Books, 2018, 47.

13 Grob, *Mental Illness and American Society,* 9, note 3.

14 David Shenk, *The Forgetting: Alzheimer's: Portrait of an Epidemic,* reprint ed. New York: Anchor, 2003.

15 "Distinguished French Alienists on General Paralysis. From the Reports of Discussions by the Medico-Psychological Society of Paris, in the *Annales Médico-Psychologiques,* 1858–59." *American Journal of Insanity,* January 1860.

16 E. Salomon, "On the Pathological Elements of General Paresis or Paresifying Mental Disease." *American Journal of Insanity* 19.4 (April 1863): 416–42.

17 Ibid.

18 A. E. Macdonald, "General Paresis." *American Journal of Insanity* 33.4 (April 1877): 451–82.

19 Allan Brandt, *No Magic Bullet: A Social History of Venereal Disease in the United States Since 1880,* enlarged ed. New York: Oxford University Press, 1987, 9.

20 Macdonald, "General Paresis."

21 R. S. Dewey, "Differentiation in Institutions for the Insane." *American Journal of Insanity* 39.1 (July 1882): 1–21.

22 Grob, *Mental Illness and American Society,* 8.
23 Ibid., 89–90.
24 Ibid., 91–92.
25 David J. Rothman, *The Discovery of the Asylum: Social Order and Disorder in the New Republic,* 2nd ed. London and New York: Routledge, 2002.

CHAPTER 4. *EXITUS LETALIS*

1 Charles K. Mills and Mary A. Schively, "Preliminary Report, Clinical and Pathological, of a Case of Progressive Dementia." *American Journal of Insanity* 54.2 (1897): 201–11.
2 William L. Russell, "Senility and Senile Dementia." *American Journal of Insanity* 58.4 (1902): 625–33.
3 Richard H. Hutchings, "The President's Address." *American Journal of Psychiatry* 96.1 (1939): 1–15.
4 Mary Kaplan and Alfred R. Henderson, "Solomon Carter Fuller, M.D. (1872–1953): American Pioneer in Alzheimer's Disease Research." *Journal of the History of the Neurosciences* 9.3 (2000): 250–61.
5 Konrad Maurer, Stephan Volk, and Hector Gerbaldo, "Auguste D: The History of Alois Alzheimer's First Case." In Peter J. Whitehouse, Konrad Maurer, and Jesse F. Ballenger, eds., *Concepts of Alzheimer Disease: Biological, Clinical and Cultural Perspectives.* Baltimore, MD: Johns Hopkins University Press, 2000, 5–29.
6 Solomon C. Fuller, "A Study of the Neurofibrils in Dementia Paralytica, Dementia Senilis, Chronic Alcoholism, Cerebral Lues and Microcephalic Idiocy." *American Journal of Insanity* 63.4 (1907): 415–68 (plus plates/figures).
7 Robert Remak's Berlin dissertation, "Vide Bethe, Allg. Anat. u. Physiol. des Nervensystems," p. 13, cited in Fuller, "Study of Neurofibrils," ref. 2.
8 Maurer, Volk, and Gerbaldo, "Auguste D," 13.
9 Alois Alzheimer, "Uber einen eigenartigen schweren Krankheitsprozess der Hirnrinde." *Zentralblatt für Nervenheilkunde und Psychiatrie* 30 (1907): 117–19.
10 Maurer, Volk, and Gerbaldo, "Auguste D," 26.
11 C. Macfie Campbell, "Arterio-Sclerosis in Relation to Mental Disease." *American Journal of Insanity* 64.3 (1908): 553–61.
12 E. E. Southard, "Anatomical Findings in Senile Dementia: A Diagnostic Study Bearing Especially on the Group of Cerebral Atrophies." *American Journal of Insanity* 66.4 (1910): 673–708.
13 Solomon C. Fuller, "Alzheimer's Disease (Senium Præcox): The Report of a Case and Review of Published Cases." *The Journal of Nervous and Mental Disease* 39.7 (1912): 440–55.
14 Solomon C. Fuller and Henry I. Klopp, "Further Observations on Alzheimer's Disease." *American Journal of Insanity* 69.1 (1912): 17–29.
15 Fuller and Klopp, "Further Observations," 27.
16 Robert Katzman and Katherine L. Bick, "The Rediscovery of Alzheimer Disease During the 1960s and 1970s." In Peter J. Whitehouse, Konrad Maurer, and Jesse F. Ballenger, eds., *Concepts of Alzheimer Disease: Biological, Clinical and Cultural Perspectives.* Baltimore, MD: Johns Hopkins University Press, 2000, 104–14.

17 Solomon C. Fuller, "A Study of the Miliary Plaques Found in Brains of the Aged." *American Journal of Insanity* 68.2 (1911): 147–220.

18 Ibid.

19 Ibid., 212.

20 David A. Snowdon, "Healthy Aging and Dementia: Findings from the Nun Study." *Annals of Internal Medicine* 139.5, pt. 2 (2003): 450–54.

21 K. Blennow et al., "Clinical Utility of Cerebrospinal Fluid Biomarkers in the Diagnosis of Early Alzheimer's Disease." *Alzheimer's and Dementia* 11.1 (2015): 58–69.

22 Adolf Meyer, "Presidential Address: Thirty-Five Years of Psychiatry in the United States and Our Present Outlook." *American Journal of Psychiatry* 85.1 (1928): 1–31.

23 Papers of Meta Vaux Warrick Fuller, Schomburg Center for Research in Black Culture, New York Public Library, file 16.

24 Mary Kaplan, *Solomon Carter Fuller: Where My Caravan Has Rested.* Lanham, MD: University Press of America, 2005.

25 Papers of Meta Vaux Warrick Fuller, Schomburg Center for Research in Black Culture, New York Public Library, file 13.

26 Rose Upton Bascom, typed manuscript titled "The Most Interesting Person in Our Town." Papers of Meta Vaux Warrick Fuller, Schomburg Center for Research in Black Culture, New York Public Library, file 12.

27 Mary Kaplan and Alfred R. Henderson, "Solomon Carter Fuller, M.D. (1872–1953): American Pioneer in Alzheimer's Disease Research." *Journal of the History of the Neurosciences* 9.3 (2000): 250–61.

CHAPTER 5. DARKNESS INTO LIGHT

1 Siddhartha Mukherjee, *The Emperor of All Maladies: A Biography of Cancer.* New York: Scribner, 2010.

2 Barron H. Lerner, *The Breast Cancer Wars: Hope, Fear, and the Pursuit of a Cure in Twentieth-Century America.* New York: Oxford University Press, 2003.

3 Adolf Meyer, "The Problem of the State in the Care of the Insane." *American Journal of Insanity* 65.4 (1909): 689–705.

4 Charles P. Bancroft, "Presidential Address: Hopeful and Discouraging Aspects of the Psychiatric Outlook." *American Journal of Insanity* 65.1 (1908): 1–16.

5 Clarence J. Gamble, "The Sterilization of Psychotic Patients Under State Laws." *American Journal of Psychiatry* 105.1 (1948): 60–62.

6 Horatio M. Pollock, "Family Care of Mental Patients." *American Journal of Psychiatry* 91.2 (1934): 331–36.

7 Jeffrey A. Lieberman, with Ogi Ogas, *Shrinks: The Untold Story of Psychiatry.* New York: Little, Brown, 2015.

8 Sylvia Nasar, *A Beautiful Mind.* New York: Simon & Schuster, 1998.

9 Elliot S. Valenstein, *Great and Desperate Cures: The Rise and Decline of Psychosurgery and Other Radical Treatments for Mental Illness.* New York: Basic Books, 1986.

10 Joshua J. Wind and D. E. Anderson, "From Prefrontal Leucotomy to Deep Brain Stimulation: The Historical Transformation of Psychosurgery and the Emergence of Neuroethics." *Neurosurgical Focus,* 25.1 (2008): E10.

11 Gerald N. Grob, *From Asylum to Community: Mental Health Policy in Modern America*. Princeton, NJ: Princeton University Press, 2014, 28.

12 Ibid., 160.

13 Gerald N. Grob, *Mental Illness and American Society, 1875–1940*. Princeton, NJ: Princeton University Press, 1983.

14 Grob, *From Asylum to Community*, 75–77.

15 Ibid., 28.

16 Grob, *Mental Illness and American Society, 1875–1940*.

17 For more on issues with deinstitutionalization, see Richard H. Lamb and Linda E. Weinberger, *Deinstitutionalization: Promise and Problems*. New York: Jossey-Bass, 2001.

18 Grob, *Mental Illness and American Society, 1875–1940*, 317, note 3.

19 Soo Borson et al., "Nursing Homes and the Mentally Ill Elderly." *A Report of the Task Force on Nursing Homes and the Mentally Ill Elderly*. Washington, DC: American Psychiatric Association, 1989.

20 Bruce C. Vladeck, *Unloving Care: The Nursing Home Tragedy*. A Twentieth Century Fund Study. New York: Basic Books, 1980.

21 Ibid., 43.

22 Ibid., 59.

23 Ibid., 56.

24 Ibid.

25 While there were virtuous for-profits and larcenous nonprofits, the strongest evidence of wrongdoing in this period emerged from the for-profit sector. Charles Hynes, *Fourth Annual Report*, Medicaid Fraud Control, New York: Office of the Special Prosecutor, 1978, p 1.

26 Ibid., 7.

27 Ibid., 12–13.

28 Ibid., 13.

29 Vladeck, *Unloving Care*, 177.

30 Ibid., 187.

31 Hynes, *Fourth Annual Report*, 53–55.

32 Ibid., 57.

33 Vladeck, *Unloving Care*, 57.

34 Jesse F. Ballenger, "Beyond the Characteristic Plaques and Tangles: Mid-Twentieth-Century U.S. Psychiatry and the Fight Against Senility." In Peter J. Whitehouse, Konrad Maurer, and Jesse F. Ballenger, eds., *Concepts of Alzheimer Disease: Biological, Clinical and Cultural Perspectives*. Baltimore, MD: Johns Hopkins University Press, 2000, 83–103.

35 Ballenger, "Beyond the Characteristic Plaques and Tangles."

36 Saul R. Korey Department of Neurology, "Remembering Saul R. Korey, M.D.: 50 Years, a Lasting Legacy." 2013; einstein.yu.edu/departments/neurology/saul-korey.aspx.

37 Robert Terry, "Neuropathologist, Electronmicroscopist, Close Collaborator: Saul Korey." einstein.yu.edu/docs/features/terry-robert-remembrance.pdf.

38 Robert Katzman and Katherine L. Bick. "The Rediscovery of Alzheimer Disease During the 1960s and 1970s." In *Concepts of Alzheimer Disease: Biological, Clinical and Cultural Perspectives*, 107.

39 Isabelle Rapin, "A History of the Saul R. Korey Department of Neurology at the Albert Einstein College of Medicine, 1955–2001." *Einstein Quarterly Journal of Biology and Medicine* 19 (2003): 68–78.

40 Peter Davies, interview by author, tape-recorded phone call, May 10, 2015.

41 Robert Katzman, "Editorial: The Prevalence and Malignancy of Alzheimer Disease. A Major Killer." *Archives of Neurology* 33.4 (1976): 217–18.

42 Katzman, "The Prevalence and Malignancy of Alzheimer Disease."

43 Peter Davies interview.

44 Nancy Dubler, interview by author, tape-recorded phone call, May 4, 2016.

45 Ronald Sullivan, "Head of Montefiore Forced to Step Down in Hospital Dispute." *New York Times*. May 9, 1985.

CHAPTER 6. PRINCESSES AND PRESIDENTS: DEMENTIA REBRANDED

1 Judith Robinson, *Noble Conspirator: Florence S. Mahoney and the Rise of the National Institutes of Health*. Washington D.C.: Francis Press, 2001. Quoted in Carla Baranauckas, "Florence S. Mahoney, 103, Health Advocate." *New York Times*. December 16, 2002.

2 Siddhartha Mukherjee, *The Emperor of All Maladies: A Biography of Cancer*. New York: Scribner, 2010.

3 Robinson, *Noble Conspirator*.

4 Ibid., 34.

5 Ibid.

6 For Merlin K. DuVal's testimony before the House Public Health and Environment Subcommittee hearings, see "Institute of Aging," *CQ Almanac 1972*, 28th ed. Washington DC: Congressional Quarterly, 1973, 03-425–03-426; library.cqpress.com /cqalmanac/document.php?id=cqal72-1250829.

7 For H. R. Gross's testimony during the House floor debate, see "Institute of Aging."

8 W. Andrew Achenbaum and Daniel M. Albert, *Profiles in Gerontology: A Biographical Dictionary*. Westport, CT: Greenwood Press, 1995. Cited in W. Andrew Achenbaum, *Robert N. Butler, MD: Visionary of Healthy Aging*. New York: Columbia University Press, 2013, 98.

9 R. L. Peck, "'A Rough Old Age'—Interview with Geriatrics Expert Robert Butler." *Nursing Homes: Long Term Management Care* (1996). Quoted in Achenbaum, *Robert N. Butler*, 74.

10 Robert N. Butler, *Why Survive? Being Old in America*. New York: Harper & Row, 1975. Quoted in Achenbaum, *Robert N. Butler*, 84.

11 Achenbaum, *Robert N. Butler*, 84.

12 Ibid., 71.

13 Butler, *Why Survive?*

14 Achenbaum, *Robert N. Butler*, 98, citing personal communication with Robert Butler, January 2, 2010.

15 Patrick Fox, "From Senility to Alzheimer's Disease: The Rise of the Alzheimer's Disease Movement." *Milbank Quarterly* 67.1 (1989): 58–102; milbank.org/quarterly /articlesfrom-senility-to-alzheimers-disease-the-rise-of-the-alzheimers-disease-move ment.

16 Zaven Khachaturian, interview by author, tape-recorded phone call, December 28, 2015.
17 Ibid.
18 Fox, "From Senility to Alzheimer's Disease."
19 Dominic Ruscio, interview by author, Washington, DC, September 15, 2016.
20 Jerome Stone, personal communication to Patrick Fox, October 30, 1986; quoted in Fox, "From Senility to Alzheimer's Disease," 80.
21 Robert Terry, letter to Jerome Stone. March 15, 1979. Katzman Archives, Special Collections and Archives, University of California–San Diego.
22 Robert Katzman, letter to Jerome Stone. May 23, 1979. Katzman Archives, University of California–San Diego.
23 Ibid.
24 Present at the meeting were, among others, Miriam Aronson from Einstein, Leopold Liss from Ohio, Anne Bashkiroff from San Francisco, Warren Easterly from Seattle, Hilda Pridgeon and Bobbie Glaze from Minnesota, and Marian Emr from NIH. Bobbie Glaze, *History of Alzheimer's Disease and Related Disorders Association*, 1983. Manuscript in Katzman Archives, University of California–San Diego.
25 Dominic Ruscio interview.
26 Ibid.
27 Dominic Ruscio and Nick Cavarocchi, *Alzheimer's Disease: Getting On the Political Agenda,* 1984. Manuscript in Katzman Archives, University of California–San Diego.
28 Katzman Archives, Special Collections & Archives, University of California–San Diego.
29 Abigail Van Buren, *Dear Abby.* Universal Press Syndicate, October 23, 1980. Article appeared in wide national syndication.
30 *Life,* April 7, 1958, 102–12.
31 "Dear Abby Creator Has Alzheimer's, Family Announces." *Chicago Tribune,* August 7, 2002.
32 Dominic Ruscio interview.
33 Ruscio and Cavarocchi. *Alzheimer's Disease: Getting On the Political Agenda.*
34 Dominic Ruscio interview.
35 Nancy L. Mace and Peter V. Rabins. *The 36-Hour Day: A Family Guide to Caring for People Who Have Alzheimer Disease, Related Dementias, and Memory Loss,* 6th ed. Baltimore, MD: Johns Hopkins University Press, 2017.
36 Lily Rothman, "Alzheimer's Awareness: What Ronald Reagan Told the World." *Time,* September 1, 2016.
37 Michael R. Gordon, "In Poignant Public Letter, Reagan Reveals That He Has Alzheimer's." *New York Times.* November 6, 1994.
38 Lawrence K. Altman, "Parsing Ronald Reagan's Words for Early Signs of Alzheimer's." *New York Times.* March 30, 2015.
39 International Medical News Service, "Marketing Is Reason for Rapid Rise in Alzheimer Research Funds." *Internal Medicine News* 18.9 (1984). Katzman Archives, University of California–San Diego.
40 Robert N. Butler, "Is the National Institute on Aging Mission Out of Balance?" *The Gerontologist* 39.4 (1999): 389–91. Web, quoted in Achenbaum, *Robert N. Butler, MD,* 98.

41 J. Grimley Evans, "Ageing and Disease." *Research and the Ageing Population: CIBA Foundation Symposium 134,* David Evered and Julie Whelan, eds. New York: John Wiley and Sons, 1988, 38–57. Quoted in Jesse Ballenger, *Self, Senility, and Alzheimer's Disease in Modern America: A History.* Baltimore, MD: Johns Hopkins University Press, 2006, 110.

42 Ballenger, *Self, Senility, and Alzheimer's Disease in Modern America,* 110; Margaret M. Lock, *The Alzheimer Conundrum: Entanglements of Dementia and Aging.* Princeton, NJ: Princeton University Press, 2013.

43 Robert Katzman, personal communication, November 1985, quoted in Fox, "From Senility to Alzheimer's Disease," 71.

44 For more on the overlap between Alzheimer's and normal aging, see Lock, *The Alzheimer Conundrum.*

CHAPTER 7. DEMENTIA'S PROGRESS

1 Review by A. F. Tredgold in *Eugenics Review* (July 19, 1927) 2.1: 34–35. Review of *Epilepsy: A Functional Illness,* by R. G. Rows and W. E. Bond.

2 For a wonderfully readable account of the evolution of neuroscience, see Eric Kandel, *In Search of Memory: The Emergence of a New Science of Mind.* New York: W. W. Norton, 2006.

3 Contemporary psychoanalysts generally embrace the insights of biological psychiatry and often incorporate medications and knowledge of genetic burden into analytically based treatments with patients. For a book-length account of how analytic practice integrates the insights of neuroscience, see Susan Vaughan, *The Talking Cure.* New York: G. P. Putnam's Sons, 1997.

4 Thomas Szasz, "The Myth of Mental Illness." *American Psychologist* 15.2 (1960): 113–18.

5 For a helpful discussion of the history of PTSD, see Jeffrey A. Lieberman, with Ogi Ogas, *Shrinks: The Untold Story of Psychiatry.* New York: Little, Brown, 2015.

6 VA/DoD Clinical Practice Guidelines, "Management of Posttraumatic Stress Disorder and Acute Stress Reaction." U.S. Department of Veterans Affairs; healthquality .va.gov/guidelines/MH/ptsd/.

7 Robert Katzman and Katherine L. Bick, "The Rediscovery of Alzheimer Disease During the 1960s and 1970s." In Peter J. Whitehouse, Konrad Maurer, and Jesse F. Ballenger, eds., *Concepts of Alzheimer Disease: Biological, Clinical and Cultural Perspectives.* Baltimore, MD: Johns Hopkins University Press, 2000, 104–14.

8 Katzman and Bick, "The Rediscovery of Alzheimer Disease During the 1960s and 1970s."

9 Stephanie J. B. Vos et al., "Modifiable Risk Factors for Prevention of Dementia in Midlife, Late Life and the Oldest-Old: Validation of the LIBRA Index." *Journal of Alzheimer's Disease* 58.2 (2017): 537–47.

10 Jesse F. Ballenger, "Beyond the Characteristic Plaques and Tangles: Mid-Twentieth Century US Psychiatry and the Fight Against Senility." *Concepts of Alzheimer Disease: Biological, Clinical, and Cultural Perspectives,* 83–103.

11 See, for instance, "Visiting the Psychiatrist," by the St. Louis chapter of the Alzheimer's Association, which includes the quote "Alzheimer's Disease is not a mental

illness"; alz.org/documents/stl/Visiting_the_Psychiatrist.pdf. Also see "One to One: Lou-Ellen Barkan, CEO and President of the Alzheimer's Association": youtube .com/watch?v=fI_6V968eZY. Interview June 2, 2011, with Sheryl McCarthy of City University, *One to One* series.

12 Lewis Thomas, *The Lives of a Cell: Notes of a Biology Watcher.* New York: Viking Press, 1974.

13 "A Timeline of HIV and AIDS," HIV.gov, updated 2016; hiv.gov/hiv-basics /overview/history/hiv-and-aids-timeline.

14 Ibid.

15 Ibid.

16 Richard L. Ernst and Joel W. Hay, "The US Economic and Social Costs of Alzheimer's Disease Revisited." *American Journal of Public Health* 84.8 (1994): 1261–64.

17 "Budget," HIV.gov, updated May 23, 2017. aids.gov/federal-resources/funding -opportunities/how-were-spending. This shows NIH research funding for HIV/ AIDS at $2.569 billion for 2016. Compare to Alzheimer's Association, "Alzheimer's Research Funding on Path to Another Historic Milestone with Announcement of $400 million Increase," 2016, alz.org/documents_custom/funding_increase _release_060616.pdf. This document cites new funding that will take NIH Alzheimer funding to just over $1 billion.

18 Alzheimer's Association, "Congress Delivers Historic Alzheimer's Research Funding Increase for Second Consecutive Year," May 1, 2017; alz.org/documents_custom /historic-funding-2017.pdf.

19 Dominic Ruscio interview.

20 Leah Klumph, "Alzheimer's: Mystery Disease of the Elderly." *CQ Editorial Research Reports* 11.18 (1983): 843.

21 Thomas, *Lives of a Cell.*

22 Meredith Wadman, "U.S. Aims for Effective Alzheimer's Treatment Strategy by 2020." *Scientific American*, 2012; scientificamerican.com/article/us-aims-effective -alzheimers-treatment-strategy-2020/.

23 Geoffrey Cowley, "Medical Mystery Tour: What Causes Alzheimer's Disease, and How Does It Ruin the Brain?" *Newsweek,* December 18, 1989: 18–89.

24 Thomas S. Kuhn, *The Structure of Scientific Revolutions*, 2nd ed. Chicago: University of Chicago Press, 1970.

25 Benjamin L. Wolozin et al., "A Neuronal Antigen in the Brains of Alzheimer Patients." *Science* 232.4750 (1986): 648–50.

26 Michael T. Heneka et al., "Neuroinflammation in Alzheimer's Disease." *The Lancet Neurology* 14.4 (2015): 388–405.

27 D. M. Bowen et al., "Neurotransmitter-Related Enzymes and Indices of Hypoxia in Senile Dementia and Other Abiotrophies." *Brain: A Journal of Neurology* 99.3 (1976): 459–96.

28 Peter Davies and A. J. Maloney, "Selective Loss of Central Cholinergic Neurons in Alzheimer's Disease." *The Lancet* 308.8000 (1976): 1403.

29 J. Wesson Ashford, "Treatment of Alzheimer's Disease: The Legacy of the Cholinergic Hypothesis, Neuroplasticity, and Future Directions." *Journal of Alzheimer's Disease* 47.1 (2015): 149–56.

30 Elaine K. Perry et al., "Necropsy Evidence of Central Cholinergic Deficits in Senile Dementia." *The Lancet* 309.8004 (1977): 189.

31 W. D. Boyd et al., "Clinical Effects of Choline in Alzheimer Senile Dementia." *The Lancet* 310.8040 (1977): 711.

32 Peter J. Whitehouse et al., "Alzheimer Disease: Evidence for Selective Loss of Cholinergic Neurons in the Nucleus Basalis." *Annals of Neurology* 10.2 (1981): 122–26.

33 William Koopmans Summers et al., "Oral Tetrahydroaminoacridine in Long-Term Treatment of Senile Dementia, Alzheimer Type." *New England Journal of Medicine* 315.20 (1986): 1241–45.

34 Kenneth L. Davis and Richard C. Mohs, "Cholinergic Drugs in Alzheimer's Disease." *New England Journal of Medicine* 315.20 (1986): 1286–87.

35 An excellent discussion of the problems with the cholinergic hypothesis and treatments based upon it is in Jesse F. Ballenger, *Self, Senility, and Alzheimer's Disease in Modern America*. Baltimore, MD: Johns Hopkins University Press, 2006, 92–101.

36 Lidia Blanco-Silvente et al., "Discontinuation, Efficacy, and Safety of Cholinesterase Inhibitors for Alzheimer's Disease: A Meta-Analysis and Meta-Regression of 43 Randomized Clinical Trials Enrolling 16,106 Patients." *International Journal of Neuropsychopharmacology* 20.7 (2017): 519–28.

37 Joe Verghese, interview by author, Bronx, New York, January 29, 2015.

CHAPTER 8. THE AMYLOID HYPOTHESIS FALLS APART

1 Jeffrey L. Cummings, Travis Morstorf, and Kate Zhong, "Alzheimer's Disease Drug-Development Pipeline: Few Candidates, Frequent Failures." *Alzheimer's Research & Therapy* 6.4 (2014): 37.

2 Hannah Devlin, "Alzheimer's Treatment Within Reach After Successful Drug Trial." *The Guardian,* November 2, 2016.

3 Michael F. Egan, James Kost, Pierre Tariot, Paul S. Aisen et al. "Randomized Trial of Verubecestat for Mild-to-Moderate Alzheimer's Disease." *New England Journal of Medicine* 378(2018): 1691–1703.

4 "The Alzheimer's Laboratory," aired November 27, 2016. cbsnews.com/news/60-minutes-alzheimers-disease-medellin-colombia-lesley-stahl/.

5 T. Fagan, "Crenezumab Disappoints in Phase 2, Researchers Remain Hopeful." Alzforum, July 22, 2014.

6 Reisa Sperling, interview by author, tape-recorded phone call, March 26, 2015.

7 Ulrike C. Müller and Hui Zheng, "Physiological Functions of APP Family Proteins." *Cold Spring Harbor Perspectives in Medicine* 2.2 (2012). a006288.

8 William H. Stoothoff and Gail V. Johnson, "Tau Phosphorylation: Physiological and Pathological Consequences." *Biochimica et Biophysica Acta (BBA)—Molecular Basis of Disease* 1739.2–3 (2005): 280–97.

9 Reisa Sperling, Elizabeth Mormino, and Keith Johnson, "The Evolution of Preclinical Alzheimer's Disease: Implications for Prevention Trials." *Neuron* 84.3 (2014): 608–22.

10 John Hardy and David Allsop, "Amyloid Deposition as the Central Event in the Aetiology of Alzheimer's Disease." *Trends in Pharmacological Science* 12.10 (1991): 383–88.

11 Donald Royall, "The 'Alzheimerization' of Dementia Research." *Journal of the American Geriatrics Society* 51.2 (2003): 277–78.

12 Daniel C. Aguirre-Acevedo et al., "Cognitive Decline in a Colombian Kindred with Autosomal Dominant Alzheimer Disease: A Retrospective Cohort Study." *JAMA Neurology* 73.4 (2016): 431–38.

13 Randall J. Bateman et al., "Autosomal Dominant Alzheimer's Disease: A Review and Proposal for the Prevention of Alzheimer's Disease." *Alzheimer's Research and Therapy* 3.1 (2011): 1.

14 Ibid.

15 Richard Mayeux, interview by author, New York, New York, February 11, 2015.

16 Miguel Calero et al., "Additional Mechanisms Conferring Genetic Susceptibility to Alzheimer's Disease." *Frontiers in Cellular Neuroscience* 9 (2015): 138.

17 Guojun Bu, "Apolipoprotein E and Its Receptors in Alzheimer's Disease: Pathways, Pathogenesis and Therapy." *Nature Reviews in Neuroscience* 10.5 (May 2009): 333–44.

18 E. H. Corder et al., "Protective Effect of Apolipoprotein E Type 2 Allele for Late Onset Alzheimer Disease." *Nature Genetics* 7.2 (1994): 180–84.

19 Yun Freudenberg-Hua et al., "Disease Variants in Genomes of 44 Centenarians." *Molecular Genetics and Genomic Medicine* 2.5 (2014): 438–50.

20 Stephen Salloway et al., "Two Phase 3 Trials of Bapineuzumab in Mild-to-Moderate Alzheimer's Disease." *New England Journal of Medicine* 370.4 (2014): 322–33; Rachelle S. Doody et al., "Phase 3 Trials of Solanezumab for Mild-to-Moderate Alzheimer's Disease." *New England Journal of Medicine* 370.4 (2014): 311–21.

21 Salloway et al., "Two Phase 3 Trials of Bapineuzumab in Mild-to-Moderate Alzheimer's Disease."

22 Doody et al., "Phase 3 Trials of Solanezumab for Mild-to-Moderate Alzheimer's Disease."

23 K. Blennow et al., "Clinical Utility of Cerebrospinal Fluid Biomarkers in the Diagnosis of Early Alzheimer's Disease." *Alzheimer's & Dementia* 11.1 (2015): 58–69.

24 Michael Gold, "Phase II Clinical Trials of Anti-B-Amyloid Antibodies: When Is Enough, Enough?" *Alzheimer's & Dementia: Translational Research & Clinical Interventions* 3.3 (2017): 402–409.

25 Jason Karlawish, "Addressing the Ethical, Policy and Social Challenges of Preclinical Alzheimer Disease." *Neurology* 77.15 (2011): 1487–93.

26 Rong Wang et al., "Incidence and Effects of Polypharmacy on Clinical Outcome among Patients Aged 80+: A Five-Year Follow-Up Study." *PLoS One* 10.11 (2015).

27 Reisa Sperling et al., "The A4 Study: Stopping AD Before Symptoms Begin?" *Science Translational Medicine* 6.228 (2014): 228.

28 Meg Tirrell, "Biogen Alzheimer's Drug Exceeds Expectations," CNBC, March 20, 2015. cnbc.com/2015/03/19/biogen-alzheimers-drug-exceeds-expectations.html.

29 Bailey Lipschultz and Rebecca Spalding. Biogen Drops After Alzheimer's Drug Trial Change Raises Concerns. *Bloomberg*. February 14, 2018. bloomberg.com/news/articles/2018-02-14/biogen-drops-after-alzheimer-s-drug-trial-change-raises-concerns.

30 "Lilly Announces Top-Line Results of Solanezumab Phase 3 Clinical Trial." Eli Lilly and Company, November 23, 2016. investor.lilly.com/releasedetail.cfm?ReleaseID =1000871.

31 M. B. Rogers, "A4 Researchers Raise Solanezumab Dosage, Lengthen the Trial." Alzforum, June 29, 2017. alzforum.org/news/research-news/a4-researchers-raise -solanezumab-dosage-lengthen-trial.

32 J. Madeleine Nash, "The New Science of Alzheimer's." *Time,* July 17, 2000.

33 Kristina Fiore and Randy Dotinga, "Aisen: Negative Anti-Amyloid Trial Confirms Amyloid Hypothesis." *MedPage Today,* December 9, 2016. medpagetoday.com /neurology/alzheimersdisease/61959.

34 David Snowdon, "Healthy Aging and Dementia: Findings from the Nun Study." *Annals of Internal Medicine* 139.5, pt 2 (2003): 450–54.

35 Lorrie Moore, "People Like That Are the Only People Here: Canonical Babbling in Peed Onk." *Birds of America: Stories.* New York: Alfred A. Knopf, 1998.

36 Gordon W. Allport, "The Functional Autonomy of Motives." *American Journal of Psychology* 50.1/4 (1937): 141–56.

37 Zaven Khachaturian, interview by author, tape-recorded phone call, December 28, 2016.

38 Yaakov Stern, "Cognitive Reserve in Ageing and Alzheimer's Disease." *Lancet Neurology* 11.11 (2012): 1106–12.

39 Kristine Yaffe, interview by author, tape-recorded phone call, February 21, 2015.

40 See also Ezekiel J. Emanuel, "Alzheimer's Anxiety." *New York Times,* November 16, 2013.

41 News release from the Alzheimer's Association International Conference 2017: Clinical Impact of Brain Amyloid PET Scans—Interim Results from the IDEAS Study, July 20, 2017. ideas-study.org/2017/07/20/interim-results-from-the-ideas -study-reported-at-aaic-2017-in-london/.

42 Reisa Sperling interview.

43 Snowdon, "Healthy Aging and Dementia."

44 Diego Iacono et al., "APOε2 and Education in Cognitively Normal Older Subjects with High Levels of AD Pathology at Autopsy: Findings from the Nun Study." *Oncotarget* 6.16 (2015): 14082–91.

45 Yaakov Stern, interview by author, New York, New York, March 4, 2015.

46 Casey N. Cook, Melissa E. Murray, and Leonard Petrucelli, "Understanding Biomarkers of Neurodegeneration: Novel Approaches to Detecting Tau Pathology." *Nature Medicine* 21.3 (2015): 219–20.

47 Reisa Sperling interview.

48 Laura T. Haas et al., "Silent Allosteric Modulation of mGluR5 Maintains Glutamate Signaling While Rescuing Alzheimer's Mouse Phenotypes." *Cell Reports* 20.1 (July 5, 2017): 76–88.

49 Joe Verghese interview.

50 Kristine Yaffe interview.

51 Reisa Sperling interview.

52 Eric B. Larson, Kristine Yaffe, and Kenneth M. Langa, "New Insights into the Dementia Epidemic." *New England Journal of Medicine* 369.24 (2013): 2275–77.

CHAPTER 9. MONEY, MONEY, MONEY

1 Amy Ehrlich, interview by author, Bronx, New York, July 29, 2015.

2 *Olmstead v. L. C.* (98-536) 527 U.S. 581 (1999) 138 F.3d 893, affirmed in part, vacated in part, and remanded; law.cornell.edu/supct/html/98-536.ZS.html.

3 Michael D. Hurd et al., "Monetary Costs of Dementia in the United States." *New England Journal of Medicine* 368 (2013): 1326–34.

4 The Scan Foundation, "Who Pays for Long-Term Care in the US?" January 2013. thescanfoundation.org/sites/default/files/who_pays_for_ltc_us_jan_2013_fs.pdf.

5 Ron Lieber, "One Woman's Slide from Middle Class to Medicaid." Your Money column. *New York Times,* July 7, 2017. nytimes.com/2017/07/07/your-money/one-womans-slide-from-the-upper-middle-class-to-medicaid.html?mcubz=0.

6 Hurd et al., "Monetary Costs of Dementia in the United States," see table 2.

7 Katherine Ornstein, Amy Kelley, Evan Bollens-Lund, and Jennifer Wolff, "A National Profile of End-of-Life Caregiving in the United States." *Health Affairs* 36.7 (2017): 1184–92.

8 Partnership Program, website of the Federal Long Term Care Insurance Program. ltcfeds.com/help/faq/miscellaneous_partnership.html.

9 Ballotpedia, New York State Budget and Finances, ballotpedia.org/New_York_state_budget_and_finances.

10 Bloomberg News, "Genworth Financial Struggling Under the Weight of Long-Term Care Costs." *Investment News,* March 3, 2015.

11 Ibid.

12 Suzanne K. Powell, "A Primer on Long-Term Care Insurance." *Professional Case Management* 18.3 (2013): 107–109; P. Doty, M. A. Cohen, J. Miller, and X. Shi, "Private Long-Term Care Insurance: Value to Claimants and Implications for Long-Term Care Financing." *Gerontologist* 50.5 (2010): 613–22; Anne T. Cramer and Gail A. Jensen, "Why Don't People Buy Long-Term Care Insurance?" *Journals of Gerontology, Series B* 61.4 (2006): S185–93; M. Meinert and P. Cole, "Should You Purchase Long-Term Care Insurance?" *Wall Street Journal,* May 14, 2012.

13 H. Gleckman, "Requiem for the CLASS Act." Health Affairs 30.12 (2011): 2231–34.

14 Health and Aging Policy Fellows website: healthandagingpolicy.org.

15 PHI, "Paying the Price: How Poverty Wages Undermine Home Care in America." February 16, 2015. https://phinational.org/resource/paying-the-price-how-poverty-wages-undermine-home-care-in-america.

16 Ibid.

17 For a moving tribute to Siegal, see chicagobears.com/news/article-1/Oldest-living-ex-Bear-passes-away/c664050e-a119-4e51-9f26-2d49a3116b67.

18 Tara Cortes, interview by author, New York, New York, October 4, 2015.

19 Maureen Conway, John Rodat, and Anne Inserra, "Cooperative Home Care Associates: A Case Study of a Sectoral Employment Development Approach." Economic Opportunities Program, Aspen Institute, February 1, 2002.

20 Noam Scheiber, "US Court Reinstates Home Care Pay Rules." *New York Times,* August 21, 2015.

21 Ai-jen Poo, with Ariane Conrad, *The Age of Dignity: Preparing for the Elder Boom in a Changing America.* New York: New Press, 2015.

22 Paula Span, "Planning to Age in Place? Find a Contractor Now." The New Old Age. *New York Times,* May 19, 2017. nytimes.com/2017/05/19/health/aging-in-place -contractors.html.

23 Paula Span, "Begin the Bidet." The New Old Age. *New York Times,* March 27, 2012.

24 Fredda Vladeck, *A Good Place to Grow Old: New York's Model for NORC Supportive Service Programs.* New York: United Hospital Fund, 2004. Available from uhfnyc .org/publications/203833.

25 Emily A. Greenfield et al., "A Tale of Two Community Initiatives for Promoting Aging in Place: Similarities and Differences in the National Implementation of NORC Programs and Villages." *Gerontologist* 53.6 (2013): 928–38.

26 Noelle Fields, K. A. Anderson, and H. Dabelko-Schoeny, "Effectiveness of Adult Day Services for Older Adults: A Review of the Literature from 2000 to 2011." *Journal of Applied Gerontology* 33.2 (2014): 130–63.

27 Ibid.

28 On Lok website, onlok.org.

29 M. D. Fretwell, J. S. Old, K. Zwan, and K. Simhadri, "The Elderhaus Program of All-Inclusive Care for the Elderly in North Carolina: Improving Functional Outcomes and Reducing Cost of Care: Preliminary Data." *Journal of the American Geriatric Society* 63.3 (2015): 578–83.

30 PACE, National Pace Association website, npaonline.org.

31 NYS Money Follows the Person Demonstration (MFP) website, health.ny.gov /health_care/medicaid/redesign/nys_money_follows_person_demonstration.htm.

32 Money Follows the Person website.

33 Joanne Lynn, interview by author, Washington, DC, September 14, 2016.

34 Ibid.

35 Ibid.

36 Joanne Lynn and Center for Elder Care and Advanced Illness, *Medicaring Communities: Getting What We Want and Need in Frail Old Age at an Affordable Price.* Altarum Institute, 2016.

37 Elizabeth H. Bradley and Lauren A. Taylor, *The American Health Care Paradox: Why Spending More Is Getting Us Less.* New York: Public Affairs, 2013.

CHAPTER 10. LABORERS OF LOVE

1 Mrs. S, interview by author, September 20, 2015.

2 Todd J. Richardson, S. J. Lee, M. Berg-Weger, and G. T. Grossberg, "Caregiver Health: Health of Caregivers of Alzheimer's and Other Dementia Patients." *Current Psychiatry Reports* 15.7 (2013): 367; D. M. Gilden et al., "Using US Medicare Records to Evaluate the Indirect Health Effects on Spouses: A Case Study in Alzheimer's Disease Patients." *BMC Health Services Research* 14 (2014): 291; Caroline Sutliffe, Clarissa Giebel, David Jolley, and David Challis, "Experience of Burden in Carers of People with Dementia on the Margins of Long-Term Care." *International Journal of Geriatric Psychiatry* (May 11, 2015). DOI: 10.1002/gps.4295.

3 Richard Schulz and S. Beach, "Caregiving as a Risk Factor for Mortality: The Caregiver Health Effects Study." *JAMA* 282.23 (1999): 2215–19.

4 Julie Bynum, "The Long Reach of Alzheimer's Disease: Patients, Practice, and Policy." *Health Affairs* 33.4 (2014): 534–40.
5 Bayley, John. *Elegy for Iris.* New York: St. Martin's Press, 1999.
6 Ibid., 266.
7 George Hodgman, *Bettyville: A Memoir.* New York: Penguin Group, 2015.
8 Carol Levine, "The Loneliness of the Long-Term Caregiver." *New England Journal of Medicine* 340.20 (1999): 1587–90.
9 Carol Levine, interview by author, New York, New York, July 28, 2015.
10 Ibid.
11 For an exception, see Hilde Lindemann Nelson and James Lindemann Nelson, *The Patient in the Family: An Ethics of Medicine and Families.* New York: Routledge, 1995.
12 Mary Mittelman, D. L. Roth, D. W. Coon, and W. E. Haley, "Sustained Benefit of Supportive Intervention for Depressive Symptoms in Caregivers of Patients with Alzheimer's Disease." *American Journal of Psychiatry* 161.5 (2004): 850–56.
13 Mary Mittelman, interview by author, recorded phone call, February 16, 2015.
14 Mary Mittelman interview, discussing this paper: K. H. Long, J. P. Moriarity, M. S. Mittelman, and S. S. Foldes, "Estimating the Potential Cost Savings from the New York University Caregiver Intervention in Minnesota." *Health Affairs* 33.4 (2014): 596–604.
15 Support group, invited observation by author, CaringKind, New York, New York, June 15, 2015.
16 Mrs. T, interview by author, September 28, 2015.
17 Ibid.
18 Mr. D, interview by author, tape-recorded phone call, January 27, 2015.

CHAPTER 11. TRY A LITTLE TENDERNESS

1 The playlist is based on the pioneering work of the Music & Memory program. See more on their website: musicandmemory.org/about/mission-and-vision.
2 An estimate of 45 percent is listed in the 2012 Alzheimer's Disease Facts and Figures, alz.org/downloads/facts_figures_2012.pdf. A lower estimate of 32 percent at age eighty-five, for Alzheimer's disease alone, not accounting for other types of dementia, can be found in L. E. Hebert et al., "Alzheimer Disease in the United States (2010 –2050) Estimated Using the 2010 Census." *Neurology* 80.19 (2013): 1778–83.
3 Marie-Christine Rousseau et al., "Quality of Life in Patients with Locked-In Syndrome: Evolution over a 6-Year Period." *Orphanet Journal of Rare Diseases* 10.88 (2015). DOI: 10.1186/s13023-015-0304-z.
4 Meet Me at MoMA, moma.org/meetme/index.
5 Kay Redfield Jamison, *An Unquiet Mind.* New York: Alfred A. Knopf, 1995.
6 G. Mitchell, B. McCormack, and T. McCance, "Therapeutic Use of Dolls for People Living with Dementia: A Critical Review of the Literature." *Dementia* 15.5 (September 2016): 976–1001.
7 H. Cioltan et al., "Variation in Use of Antipsychotic Medications in Nursing Homes in the US: A Systematic Review." *BMC Geriatrics* 17.1 (January 26, 2017): 32.

8 Anne Tergesen and Miho Inada, "It's Not a Stuffed Animal, It's a $6,000 Dollar Medical Device." *Wall Street Journal,* June 21, 2010.

9 Jeremy D. Larson, "Letter of Recommendation: Hasbro Joy for All." *New York Times,* March 24, 2016. nytimes.com/2016/03/27/magazine/letter-of-recommendation-hasbro-joy-for-all.html?mcubz=0.

10 Music & Memory website: musicandmemory.org/about/mission-and-vision.

11 A clip from the film is available on YouTube here: youtube.com/watch?v=fyZQf0 p73QM.

12 Singing for the Brain, Alzheimer's Society. alzheimers.org.uk/info/20172/your_support _services/765/singing_for_the_brain.

13 Alzheimer's.net Blog, "5 Reasons Why Music Boosts Brain Activity," July 21, 2014. alzheimers.net/2014-07-21/why-music-boosts-brain-activity-in-dementia-patients.

14 Joe Verghese et al., "Leisure Activities and the Risk of Dementia in the Elderly." *New England Journal of Medicine* 348 (2003): 2508–16.

15 Canada's National Ballet School and Baycrest Centre for Geriatric Care, "Movement to Music at Baycrest," nbs-enb.ca/Sharing-Dance/Sharing-Dance-Programs /Movement-to-Music-at-Baycrest.

16 Jed A. Levine, interview by author, New York, New York, October 19, 2015.

17 UK Design Council, "Living Well with Dementia," February 18, 2015. designcoun cil.org.uk/resources/case-study/living-well-dementia.

18 Dementia Dog Project, dementiadog.org.

19 Stephen G. Post, *The Moral Challenge of Alzheimer Disease.* Second edition. Baltimore, MD: Johns Hopkins University Press, 2000.

20 Tom Kitwood, *Dementia Reconsidered: The Person Comes First.* Glasgow: Open University Press, 1997.

21 Ibid., 5.

22 John Zeisel, *I'm Still Here: A New Philosophy of Alzheimer's Care.* New York: Avery, 2009.

23 John Zeisel and Paul Raia, "Non-Pharmacological Treatment for Alzheimer's Disease: A Mind-Brain Approach." *American Journal of Alzheimer's Disease and Other Dementias* 15.6 (2000): 331–40.

24 Ibid.

25 Ibid.

26 Jennifer Watson et al., "Obstacles and Opportunities in Alzheimer's Clinical Trial Recruitment." *Health Affairs* 33.4 (2014): 574–79.

27 You can learn more about the Brain Health Registry by visiting their website at brainhealthregistry.org.

28 A full description of the MindCrowd study is available on their website at mind crowd.org.

29 Henry K. Beecher, "Ethics and Clinical Research." *New England Journal of Medicine* 274.24 (1966): 1354–60.

30 See David J. Rothman, *Strangers at the Bedside: A History of How Law and Bioethics Transformed Medical Decision Making.* New York: Basic Books, 1991.

31 E. F. Scanlon, R. A. Hawkins, W. W. Fox, and W. S. Smith, "Fatal Homotransplanted Melanoma: A Case Report." *Cancer* 18 (1965): 782–89. Cited in Rothman, *Strangers at the Bedside*, appendix, 265.

32 Pam Belluck, "Sex, Dementia, and a Husband on Trial at 78." *New York Times,* April 14, 2015.

33 Atul Gawande, *Being Mortal: Medicine and What Matters in the End.* New York: Henry Holt, 2014.

34 D. Herbenick et al., "Women's Use and Perceptions of Commercial Lubricants: Prevalence and Characteristics in a Nationally Representative Sample of American Adults." *J Sex Med.* 11.3 (2014): 642–52.

35 M. Bauer et al., "'We Need to Know What's Going On': Views of Family Members Toward the Sexual Expression of People with Dementia in Residential Aged Care." *Dementia* 13.5 (2014): 571–85.

36 "Policies and Procedures Concerning Sexual Expression at the Hebrew Home at River-dale." static1.squarespace.com/static/5520af09e4b0c878b5733095/t/56328f20e4b04 afbbe92827d/1446154016232/sexualexpressionpolicy.pdf. Last revised April 2013.

37 James M. Wilkins, "More Than Capacity: Alternatives for Sexual Decision Making for Individuals with Dementia." *The Gerontologist.* 55.5 (2015): 716–23.

38 Y. J. Kim et al., "An International Comparative Study on Driving Regulations on People with Dementia." *Journal of Alzheimer's Disease* 56.3 (2017): 1007–14.

39 D. B. Carr and B. R. Ott, "The Older Adult Driver with Cognitive Impairment: 'It's a Very Frustrating Life.'" *JAMA* 303.16 (2010): 1632–42.

40 D. J. Cox et al., "Evaluating Driving Performance of Outpatients with Alzheimer Disease." *Journal of the American Board of Family Practice* 11.4 (1998): 264–71. Cited in Carr and Ott, "The Older Adult Driver with Cognitive Impairment."

41 Daniel C. Marson, "Clinical and Ethical Aspects of Financial Capacity in Dementia: A Commentary." *American Journal of Geriatric Psychiatry* 21.4 (2013): 382–90.

42 Eric Widera, Veronika Steenpass, Daniel Marson, and Rebecca Sudore, "Finances in the Older Patient with Cognitive Impairment." *JAMA* 305.7 (2011): 698–706.

43 National Committee for the Prevention of Elder Abuse. *The Metlife Study of Elder Financial Abuse: Crimes of Occasion, Desperation, and Predation Against America's Elders.* Westport, CT: Virginia Tech Metlife Mature Market Institute, 2011. metlife .com/assets/cao/mmi/publications/studies/2011/mmi-elder-financial-abuse.pdf. Cited in R. N. Spreng, J. Karlawish, and D. C. Marson, "Cognitive, Social and Neural Determinants of Diminished Decision-Making and Financial Exploitation Risk in Aging and Dementia: A Review and New Model." *Journal of Elder Abuse and Neglect* 28.4–5 (2016): 320–44.

44 Spreng, Karlawish, and Marson, "Cognitive, Social and Neural Determinants."

45 Geraldine Boyle, "She's Usually Quicker Than the Calculator: Financial Management and Decision-Making in Couples Living with Dementia." *Health and Social Care in the Community* 21.5 (2013): 554–62.

46 Marson, "Clinical and Ethical Aspects."

47 Spreng, Karlawish, and Marson, "Cognitive, Social and Neural Determinants."

48 J. J. Arias, "A Time to Step In: Legal Mechanisms for Protecting Those with Declining Capacity." *American Journal of Law and Medicine* 39.1 (2013): 134–59.

49 Consumer Financial Protection Bureau, "Recommendations and Report for Financial Institutions on Preventing and Responding to Elder Financial Exploitation."

files.consumerfinance.gov/f/201603_cfpb_recommendations-and-report-for-financial
-institutions-on-preventing-and-responding-to-elder-financial-exploitation.pdf.

50 CFPB, "Recommendations."

CHAPTER 12. A GOOD ENDING

1 James Hallenbeck et al., The Stanford Faculty Development Center End-of-Life Care Curriculum for Medical Teachers. 2003. growthhouse.org/stanford/elc _handbook_v181.pdf.

2 National Center for Health Statistics, "Trends in Inpatient Hospital Deaths: National Hospital Discharge Survey, 2000–2010." Centers for Disease Control and Prevention. cdc.gov/nchs/products/databriefs/db118.htm.

3 Melissa Wachterman, Dan K. Kiely, and Susan L. Mitchell, "Reporting Dementia on the Death Certificates of Nursing Home Residents Dying with End-Stage Dementia."*JAMA* 300.22 (2008): 2608–10.

4 B. Reisberg, S. H. Ferris, M. J. de Leon, and T. Crook, "The Global Deterioration Scale for Assessment of Primary Degenerative Dementia." *American Journal of Psychiatry* 139.9 (1982): 1136–39.

5 Susan Mitchell et al., "The Clinical Course of Advanced Dementia." *New England Journal of Medicine* 361.16 (2009): 1529–38.

6 Ibid.

7 J. R. Lunney et al., "Patterns of Functional Decline at the End of Life." *Journal of the AMA* 289.18 (2003): 2387–92.

8 Melissa Aldridge and Elizabeth Bradley, "Epidemiology and Patterns of Care at the End of Life: Rising Complexity, Shifts in Care Patterns, and Sites of Death." *Health Affairs* 36.7 (2017): 1175–83.

9 Julia Driessen and Turner West, "Variation in End-of-Life Care Is an Open Invitation for Accountable Care Organization Innovation." Health Affairs Blog, August 25, 2017; healthaffairs.org/blog/2017/08/25/variation-in-end-of-life-care-is-an -open-invitation-for-accountable-care-organization-innovation.

10 Terri R. Fried et al., "Understanding the Treatment Preferences of Seriously Ill Patients." *New England Journal of Medicine* 346.14 (2002): 1061–66.

11 Henry S. Perkins, "Controlling Death: The False Promise of Advance Directives." *Annals of Internal Medicine* 147.1 (2007): 51–57.

12 Here I summarize sketchily some hundreds of articles and thirty-five years of scholarly work. For key readings on this topic, see Ronald Dworkin, *Life's Dominion: An Argument About Abortion, Euthanasia, and Individual Freedom.* New York: Alfred A. Knopf, 1993; and Rebecca Dresser and P. Whitehouse, "The Incompetent Patient on the Slippery Slope." *Hastings Center Report* 24.4 (1994): 6–12.

13 Pedro Gozalo et al., "End-of-Life Transitions Among Nursing Home Residents with Cognitive Issues." *New England Journal of Medicine* 365 (2011): 1212–21.

14 J. A. Tulsky et al., "A Research Agenda for Communication Between Health Care Professionals and Patients Living with Serious Illness." *JAMA Internal Medicine* 177.9 (2017): 1361–66.

15 Susan L. Mitchell, "Advanced Dementia." *New England Journal of Medicine* 376.26 (2015): 2533–40. E. L. Sampson, B. Candy, and L. Jones, "Enteral Tube Feeding for Older People with Advanced Dementia." *Cochrane Database of Systematic Reviews* 2 (2009): CD007209.

16 American Geriatrics Society, "Choosing Wisely," an Initiative of the ABIM Foundation. choosingwisely.org/societies/american-geriatrics-society/.

17 Paul T. Menzel and Colette Chandler-Cramer, "Advance Directives, Dementia and Withholding Food and Water by Mouth." *Hastings Center Report* 44.3 (2014): 23–37.

18 D. R. Cooley, "A Kantian Moral Duty for the Soon-to-Be Demented to Commit Suicide." *American Journal of Bioethics* 7.6 (2007): 37–44.

19 Tia Powell and Adrienne Asch, "A Modest Proposal for Reducing Imperfection and Resolving World Hunger." *American Journal of Bioethics* 7.6 (2007): 53–55.

20 Robin Marantz Henig, "The Last Day of Her Life." *New York Times.* May 14, 2015; nytimes.com/2015/05/17/magazine/the-last-day-of-her-life.html?mcubz=0.

21 C. O. Long, "Pain Management Education in Long-Term Care: It Can Make a Difference." *Pain Management Nursing* 14.4 (December 2013): 220–27.

22 CaringKind, "Palliative Care for People with Dementia." CaringKind, 2016.

23 Ibid., example on 20–21.

24 Stephen G. Post, *The Moral Challenge of Alzheimer Disease: Ethical Issues from Diagnosis to Dying.* Baltimore, MD: Johns Hopkins University Press, 2000.

25 A Place for Mom: Connecting Families to Senior Living, aplaceformom.com/senior-care-resources/cost-of-care.

26 Paula Span, *When the Time Comes: Families with Aging Parents Share Their Struggles and Solutions.* New York: Grand Central Life and Style, 2009.

Index